GESTATIONAL D COOKBOOK

Tasty and easy recipes with pregnancy-friendly food & 28- day meal plan that won't make you fear for your baby's health
You and your baby will no longer be alone!

Samantha Smyth

© Copyright 2021 - All rights reserved. This document is geared towards providing exact and reliable information in regard to the topic and issue covered. - From a Declaration of Principles which was accepted and approved equally by a Committee of the American Bar Association and a Committee of Publishers and Associations. In no way is it legal to reproduce, duplicate, or transmit any part of this document in either electronic means or in printed format. All rights reserved. The information provided herein is stated to be truthful and consistent, in that any liability, in terms of inattention or otherwise, by any usage or abuse of any policies, processes, or directions contained within is the solitary and utter responsibility of the recipient reader. Under no circumstances will any legal responsibility or blame be held against the publisher for any reparation, damages, or monetary loss due to the information herein, either directly or indirectly. Respective authors own all copyrights not held by the publisher. The information herein is offered for informational purposes solely and is universal as so. The presentation of the information is without contract or any type of guarantee assurance. The trademarks that are used are without any consent, and the publication of the trademark is without permission or backing by the trademark owner. All trademarks and brands within this book are for clarifying purposes only and are owned by the owners themselves, not affiliated with this document.

This book is intended solely for informational and educational purposes and not personal medical advice. Always seek the advice of your physician with any questions you have regarding a medical condition, and before undertaking any diet, exercise, or other health program.

The information in this book is not intended to treat, diagnose, cure, or prevent any disease. The approach proposed in this book is not sponsored, recommended, or endorsed by any organization.

The author accepts no liability of any kind for any damages caused or alleged to be caused, directly or indirectly, from use of the information in this book.

TABLE OF CONTENTS

Introduction 8

Chapter 1: What to Do After Delivery to Prevent Type 2 Diabetes 10

    What Happens After Birth? 10

    What is Gestational Diabetes? 10

    How Reduce the Likelihood You'll Need Insulin By 50%? 10

    Why Is Maintaining Normal Blood Sugar So Important? 11

    Are You at Risk of Getting Gestational Diabetes? 11

Chapter 2: Diabetes Therapy 13

    Why Conventional Diet Therapy Often Fails? 13

    What Is the Diabetes Therapy? 13

    How Is Gestational Diabetes Dealt With? 14

Chapter 3: When Convention Therapy Has Failed, What Should You Do 15

Chapter 4: How to Reduce the Likelihood You'll Need Insulin by 50%. 17

Chapter 5: Foods that Will Help the Infant to Get the Right Nutrients for Optimal Development 19

Chapter 6: Foods that Raise Your Blood Sugar and Foods that Don't Raise Your Blood Sugar 21

    What Do I Need to Eat If I Actually Have Gestational Diabetes? 21

    What Complications Are Related to Gestational Diabetes? 21

    What Is the Outlook for Gestational Diabetes? 22

    Can Gestational Diabetes Be Prevented? 22

Chapter 7: Meal Timing and Spacing 23

    How Is Gestational Diabetes Controlled? 23

    When to Eat? 23

    Meal Spacing 23

    What Should I Eat? 24

    Foods to Avoid 24

Chapter 8: Food Meal Plan 25

Chapter 9: Breakfast 26

1. Berry Almond Smoothie 26
2. Tropical Greek Yogurt Bowl 27
3. Peanut Butter Power Oats 28
4. Blueberry Coconut Breakfast Cookies 29
5. Simple Grain-Free Biscuits 30
6. Orange Muffins 31
7. Crepe Cakes 32
8. Coconut Pancakes 33
9. Loaded Avocado 34
10. Breakfast Tacos 35
11. Huevos Rancheros Remix 37
12. Brussels Sprouts and Egg Scramble 38
13. Sausage, Sweet Potato, and Kale Hash 39
14. Maple Sausage Frittata 40
15. Coconut-Berry Sunrise Smoothie 41
16. Avocado and Goat Cheese Toast 42
17. Oat and Walnut Granola 43
18. Chocolate-Zucchini Muffins 44
19. Gluten-Free Carrot and Oat Pancakes 45
20. Breakfast Egg Bites 46
21. Spinach, Artichoke, and Goat Cheese Breakfast Bake 47
22. Crispy Breakfast Pita With Egg and Canadian Bacon 48
23. Brussels Sprout Hash and Eggs 49

Chapter 10: Lunch 50

24. Shrimp Paella 50
25. Salmon and Pesto Salad 51
26. Baked Fennel and Garlic Sea Bass 52
27. Lemon, Garlic, and Cilantro Tuna and Rice 53
28. Cod and Green Bean Risotto 54
29. Mixed Pepper Stuffed River Trout 55
30. Haddock and Buttered Leeks 56
31. Thai Spiced Halibut 57

32. Homemade Tuna Niçoise 58
33. Monkfish Curry 59
34. Salad With Vinaigrette 60
35. Salad With Lemon Dressing 61
36. Shrimp With Salsa 62
37. Cauliflower Soup 63
38. Cabbage Stew 64
39. Baked Haddock 65
40. Herbed Chicken 66
41. Pesto Pork Chops 67
42. Vegetable Curry 68
43. Grilled Steak With Salsa 69
44. Persian Chicken 70
45. Creamy Chicken With Cider 71
46. Exotic Palabok 72
47. Vegetarian Gobi Curry 73

Chapter 11: Snacks 74

48. Peanut Butter Sandwich Snacks 74
49. Peanut Butter Apple Slices 75
50. Baked Plantains 76
51. Strawberries and Cream Chocolate Cookie Sandwich 77
52. Mini Chocolate Chip Cookies 78
53. Chocolate-Peppermint Thins 79
54. Chocolate-Dipped Baby Bananas 80
55. Fall Harvest Salad 81
56. Two-Ingredient Ice Cream Cupcake Bites 82
57. Lemon Blueberry Cheesecake Yogurt Bark 83
58. Dark Chocolate Avocado Mousse 84
59. Hearty Chia and Blackberry Pudding 85
60. Special Cocoa Brownie Bombs 86
61. Gentle Blackberry Crumble 87
62. Mini Minty Happiness 88
63. Astonishing Maple Pecan Bacon Slices 89

64. Generous Maple and Pecan Bites 90
65. Carrot Ball Delight 91
66. Awesome Brownie Muffins 92
67. Spice Friendly Muffins 93
68. Lime Grilled Pineapple 94
69. Sherry Hummus 95
70. Fruit Potpourri 96
71. Citrus Fruit Salsa 97

Chapter 12: Dinner 98

72. Apple Glazed Chicken With Spinach 98
73. BBQ Ranch Wraps 100
74. BLT Cups 101
75. Baked Beans With Ground Beef 102
76. Baked Chicken Taquitos 103
77. Baked Fish Tacos With Avocado 104
78. Beef and Vegetables in Peanut Sauce 105
79. Black Bean Queso Wraps 106
80. Broccoli and Cauliflower Sauté 108
81. Buffalo Deviled Eggs 109
82. Cajun Shrimp Grill Packets With Tomatoes Okra 110
83. Chicken Spring Vegetable Tortellini Salad 111
84. Chicken Honey Nut Stir Fry 112
85. Curried Chicken With Cabbage, Apple and Onion 113
86. Curried Turkey Cutlets With Dried Apricots 114
87. Easy Butternut Squash Soup 115
88. Easy Deviled Eggs 116
89. Easy Grilled Zucchini 117
90. Farfalle With Tuna, Lemon, and Fennel 118
91. Fresh Sweet Corn Salad 119
92. Fresh Tomato Soup 120
93. Garlic Brussels Sprout Chips 121
94. Grapefruit Mint Chicken 122
95. Green Veggie Bowl With Chicken Lemon Tahini Dressing 123

Chapter 13: Drinks 125
- 96. Avocado Blueberry Smoothie 125
- 97. Vegan Blueberry Smoothie 126
- 98. Berry Peach Smoothie 127
- 99. Cantaloupe Blackberry Smoothie 128
- 100. Cantaloupe Kale Smoothie 129
- 101. Mix Berry Cantaloupe Smoothie 130
- 102. Avocado Kale Smoothie 131
- 103. Apple Kale Cucumber Smoothie 132
- 104. Refreshing Cucumber Smoothie 133
- 105. Cauliflower Veggie Smoothie 134
- 106. Sweet Dream Strawberry Smoothie 135
- 107. Apple Blueberry Smoothie 136
- 108. Avocado Mixed Smoothie 137
- 109. Peach Berry Smoothie 138
- 110. Irish Sea Moss Smoothie 139
- 111. Strawberry Banana Smoothie 140
- 112. Green Monster Smoothie 141
- 113. Apple Smoothie 142
- 114. Apple Cucumber Smoothie 143
- 115. Multiple Berries Smoothie 144
- 116. Kale Smoothie 145
- 117. Raspberry Smoothie 146
- 118. Pineapple Smoothie 147
- 119. Beet Smoothie 148
- 120. Blueberry Smoothie 149

Chapter 14: Prenatal Exercise 150
- Is It Safe to Exercise When You Are Pregnant? 150
- Benefits of Exercise During Pregnancy 150
- Recommended Exercise 151
- Exercises to Avoid 151

Conclusion 152

Introduction

Gestational diabetes is a type of diabetes that starts during pregnancy. It begins to develop when the body's insulin level changes to match the baby's needs. It can be hard to control and sometimes requires continuous monitoring by a doctor or midwife. The treatment for gestational diabetes is mainly focused on nutritional guidance, weight management, and oral medications. Gestational diabetes used to be called "gestational diabetes mellitus" (GDM).

Pregnant women should watch what they eat because gestational diabetes can affect their babies. Too much sugar in the blood can make the baby grow too big and put a lot of stress on the body. Babies who are born with too much sugar in their blood have an increased risk for problems during delivery and after birth. These problems include breathing trouble, jaundice, and being dehydrated. If babies get too much sugar in their system from mom's blood, it could hurt them for about a month or so after they're born. Pregnant women need to follow a diet that limits the amount of sugar they eat. They shouldn't eat large amounts of sugary foods, such as candy, cookies, cakes, and soda. Eating too much sugar can raise the amount of sugar in the blood by throwing off the balance between insulin and glucose. This will cause the baby to go into a diabetic coma which can be deadly!

You should begin taking insulin about 6 weeks before you're due to give birth. If you haven't been pregnant before, then you might not need insulin. Your healthcare provider will assist you in choosing if it's right for you.

To help control your diabetes during pregnancy, keep track of your blood sugar levels on a regular basis. This means checking your sugar before and after each meal. You should check your blood sugar again 2 hours after eating. Try not to eat more than 18 g. of carbohydrates per meal. That means you should not have more than 6 crackers, 3 sodas, or a small bowl of cereal at any one time.

When you're following a meal plan, there will be times when you will need to add insulin or oral medications to help keep your blood sugar at the right level. You should only use this type of medication when instructed by your doctor or midwife, or if the plan calls for it.

The meal plan includes a list of food items that you should eat, as well as recipes for breakfast, lunch, dinner, and snacks. You will also get information about proper nutrition, how to read food labels, food identification photos, and suitable portions of what to eat. About half the foods listed in this book are low in carbohydrates or sugar. The other half of your diet is meant to be used as a substitute for carbohydrates or sugar that you need to limit in your diet. Some examples are cheese and nuts. These can help you manage your blood sugar level without raising it too high.

This book contains the basics of Gestational Diabetes and 120 recipes that will help you manage your blood sugar while you are pregnant. It also provides information about proper nutrition, how to read food labels, and correct portions of what to eat.

Chapter 1: What to Do After Delivery to Prevent Type 2 Diabetes

What Happens After Birth?

If you were on diabetes medication, this would stop after your baby is born, under normal circumstances, and this is attributed to the fact that for most women who have gestational diabetes, blood sugar levels return to normal after delivery.

Something very important to point out is that just because you have gestational diabetes does not mean that your baby is going to be born with diabetes, but they have an increased chance of developing type 2 diabetes later in life. Another thing is that it also puts you at an increased risk of getting type 2 diabetes, and you should therefore continue watching your diet and eating whole complex carbs in place of simple, refined carbs.

What is Gestational Diabetes?

Gestational diabetes is a temporary condition that affects how your body processes sugar. You're only at risk for gestational diabetes if you have an existing diagnosis of type 2 diabetes and are currently pregnant.

Symptoms vary from person to person, but the most common signs are excessive thirst and hunger, constantly feeling thirsty or needing to pee before meals, high blood glucose levels after meals, weight gain in pregnancy or increased fat around the abdomen (sometimes with no change in weight), waking up several times per night; headaches, back pain, and blurred vision. The implications of gestational diabetes are wide-reaching and can lead to medical complications like pre-eclampsia or other serious issues for both the mother as well as the baby.

How Reduce the Likelihood You'll Need Insulin By 50%?

In type 2 diabetes, the problem is not enough insulin, whereas, in gestational diabetes, there is too much insulin flowing through the body. To prevent this, you need to be aware of the food that increases insulin, release and avoid these.

In the first trimester, it is all about protein and fats; in the second trimester, it is all about starchy carbs; and in the third trimester, it's all about fat. There are some good guidelines to help you keep track of your diet in a simple way:

Whole-food meals are essential as they are less likely to cause a spike in blood sugar levels after eating.

For example, the sugar found in processed foods and drinks has a rapid effect on blood sugar levels, while a whole-food meal rich in protein and fiber will take longer for your blood sugar level to rise after eating. For example, whole-wheat bread from a bakery is better than white bread from the supermarket. As a general rule, avoid anything white as it's stripped of its nutrients. The same goes for pasta; switch to whole-grain and use more legumes and vegetables instead.

Rice is not part of the healthy carb group because it can spike glucose levels just as much as white bread, so try basmati rice or brown rice instead.

Why Is Maintaining Normal Blood Sugar So Important?

Normal blood sugar levels can be controlled with insulin to help your body process glucose or sugar. When blood sugar is normal, the amount of insulin you need is much smaller than what you need when your blood sugar is unstable or high. The longer you've been diabetic, the greater the risk that the body will produce too much insulin in response to a high-carbohydrate meal. This leads to a burst of high blood sugars after eating when that happens, insulin levels stay elevated in the body for hours and cause hyperglycemia (excess glucose) and hypoglycemia (lowered glucose).

Are You at Risk of Getting Gestational Diabetes?

You may be at risk if:

1. Your family has a history of type 2 diabetes
2. Are 40 years old and above
3. Have had gestational diabetes in earlier pregnancies
4. Have delivered a baby weighing 4.5kg and more before
5. Are obese or overweight
6. You have (PCOS) Polycystic Ovarian Syndrome
7. You have experienced complicated pregnancies before

Now that you are equipped with the right information regarding gestation diabetes, you can now move forward confidently knowing what you should do if you have gestational diabetes or if you develop it. Below are tasty recipes designed to help balance and normalize your blood sugar levels. They are not just restricted to gestational diabetes; you can enjoy them long after birth to help you stay healthy and well-nourished.

Chapter 2: Diabetes Therapy

Diabetes is a condition that affects millions of people worldwide. Often, diabetes care is limited to diet modification without drug treatment, which often fails. This will explain some of the reasons why conventional diet therapy often fails.

Why Conventional Diet Therapy Often Fails?

The fundamental problem with conventional diet therapy is that it takes the body's metabolism for granted and attempts to control it by reducing insulin output and increasing caloric intake; the body's own metabolic controllers are ignored.
But the human body is unique among animals in its ability to maintain a constant internal environment; so, it must have evolved a special internal signaling network for that purpose. The complex system of neural, hormonal, and neutrally-mediated hormonal signals must work together to maintain the proper level of sugar in the blood.

What Is the Diabetes Therapy?

Diabetes therapy is based on the discoveries made more than a century ago by Theodor Escherich. He discovered that the hormone glucagon was secreted from the duodenal glands of animals in response to an increased level of sugar in the blood and was able to "fine-tune" the circulating level of sugar through this hormone. Using this system, he successfully used injections of glucagon to correct diabetes in humans for more than 15 years, long before the discovery that insulin was involved in diabetes.
Diabetes Therapy is based on these findings and has been demonstrated to be highly effective.
Diabetes Therapy is a new treatment for diabetes based on physiology. The therapy consists of two treatments: an injection of glucagon and ingestion of an easily absorbed carbohydrate.
These simple treatments involve only two steps:
Step 1: Glucagon Injection
This involves an injection of glucagon serum into a vein, which is absorbed by the bloodstream and taken to the liver, where it triggers a cascade of chemical reactions which leads to the following events:
- Blood sugar rises.
- Glucagon hormone levels increase in the blood plasma.
- The liver begins producing insulin.

- The liver's insulin begins to act on cells that are insulin-resistant (liver cells).
- Insulin converts excess glucose into glycogen. (This is why an injection of glucagon causes blood sugar to rise.)

Step 2: Carbohydrate Ingestion

This involves ingestion of a concentrated carbohydrate such as white bread, plantains, potatoes or rice, etc., which is absorbed by the small intestine and transported to the liver. The liver begins producing large amounts of insulin (note: this is nearly a seven-fold increase in insulin levels), which goes to the cells that are insulin-resistant to induce glucose uptake and glycogen production.

The insulin, not being able to enter the cells, becomes bound to proteins and enters the bloodstream. The effect of this is that it does not activate the same cascade of chemical reactions as does glucagon, and therefore no additional glucose is produced.

These two steps work together to balance glucose in the blood through the action of glucagon and to maintain that balance by preventing the loss of glucose by stimulating the production of glucose in the liver.

The treatment has been called "Glucagon Balancing" because it balances circulating levels of glucagon with those of insulin. This allows physiological control over blood glucose to return to normal.

How Is Gestational Diabetes Dealt With?

If you're recognized with gestational diabetes, your treatment plan will depend on your blood sugar levels at some stage in the day. In most instances, your physician will recommend you to check your blood sugar earlier than and after meals and manipulate your circumstance with the aid of eating healthy and exercising regularly. In some instances, they may additionally upload insulin injections if needed. According to the Mayo Clinic, the simplest 10-20% of girls with gestational diabetes need insulin to assist in manipulating their blood sugar. If your doctor encourages you to display your blood sugar tiers, they may supply you with a special glucose-monitoring tool. They can also prescribe insulin injections for you until you give birth. Ask your physician about nicely timing your insulin injections in terms of your food and exercise to keep away from low blood sugar. Your doctor also can inform you what to do if your blood sugar levels fall too low or are continually better than they should be.

Chapter 3: When Convention Therapy Has Failed, What Should You Do

Sometimes, conventional diet therapy fails to maintain normal blood sugar levels and insulin injections are needed. When this happens, the mother's health is at risk because of the increased risks of nutrient and oxygen deprivation to the fetus. This article will discuss gestational diabetes (GD), its causes, symptoms, diagnosis, and treatment options.

Gestational diabetes mellitus (GDM) is a type of diabetes that can start or worsen during pregnancy in some women. It is a temporary condition that usually goes away after childbirth, but it can increase your risk for type 2 diabetes later in life too.

Only pregnant women who are not diabetic may develop GDM.

You may have GDM if you have any of the following:

- The first signs of GD usually appear 2–3 weeks after conception. Your blood sugar level is determined by a fasting plasma glucose test, which is done on a sample taken from you at the doctor's office or lab. Other tests for assessing blood sugar levels, such as an oral glucose tolerance test (OGTT), may be performed as well.

Treatment for GDM is generally centered around diet and exercise modification. The goal is to keep your blood sugar level under control, preventing complications from affecting the fetus and you.

When conventional diet therapy fails, you may try the following:

If you are diabetic, you should not attempt to stop taking any of your diabetes medications until the baby is born. Your blood sugar must be monitored during pregnancy through weekly home glucose checks.

Diabetic women should take extra care when they become pregnant, especially if they have previously been diagnosed with GDM. During pregnancy, it is important to carefully monitor blood sugar levels. After childbirth, this responsibility continues. Women who are diabetic and not breastfeeding while pregnant may need an insulin pump or infusion pump during labor and delivery. Women who are taking insulin will need a continuous glucose monitor (CGM), which continuously monitors their blood sugar levels throughout the day.

GDM is a common condition, occurring in about 2–10% of pregnancies in the United States. It has been associated with an increased risk for birth defects, including congenital anomalies and neural tube defects. Women with GDM require special care during pregnancy and delivery to avoid developing further medical complications.

The complications are not usually present if the woman maintains normal blood sugar levels. The major cause of death in both the mother and baby is from a lack of oxygen during delivery. Although this can be prevented, it is a complex issue that requires careful monitoring by medical professionals.

GDM can be treated with exercise and diet modification so long as the mother maintains a healthy body weight prior to becoming pregnant.

Modifications in diet and lifestyle, as well as insulin therapy when necessary, are the cornerstones of management for pregnant women with GDM. The ADA now recommends that women with GDM aim for a 5–10% weight loss in their pregnancy (as opposed to 20% previously). This can help prevent the onset of type 2 diabetes later in life.

Dr. Bahram Arjmandi, an associate professor and head of Florida State University's nutrition department, has some advice for women with GDM. "If you have gestational diabetes, you should not attempt to lose 20%," he said. "That can cause complications in the baby, including premature birth. Instead, women should try to lose between 5–10% of their prepregnancy body weight," Arjmandi said.

Chapter 4: How to Reduce the Likelihood You'll Need Insulin by 50%

To reduce the likelihood of insulin by 50%, you shall consume 50 g. of fiber per day.
How Much Fiber Is in Your Diet?
It is recommended by the USDA that adults consume 25–35 g. of dietary fiber per day. This amount is equivalent to 1-½ to 3 cups of oatmeal, 2–3 servings of vegetables, and 3/4 cup high-quality cereal per day. Most Americans consume only about 14 g. at a time because processed foods tend to be low in fiber, and they don't include natural sugars or nutrients such as protein, calcium, or iron that lead to hunger or other unpleasant feelings like fatigue.

The most important source of dietary fiber is whole-grain products. For example, 1 cup of cooked brown rice contains 11 g. of fiber (most whole grains are high in fiber). The same is true for corn and wheat flours that result in more than 10 g. of fiber from cornmeal and many more from wheat flour, respectively.

Choose foods high in fiber like fruits, vegetables, beans, brown rice, and whole-grain bread. These are low in calories, so they help reduce your food intake. You can also add seconds to your meal when you are full to account for those extra calories that stimulate appetite. This can eliminate weight loss because your BMR is affected.

Eat breakfast that contains protein and fiber. The fiber will help improve the digestive system and will make you feel full. Eat a combination of carbohydrates, protein, and fat in your meals to ensure adequate levels of all three nutrients. You can also add an extra serving of vegetables to your meal plan. Vegetables are high in minerals, vitamins, fiber, and water which are key to keeping the body hydrated and functioning optimally.

Dietary fiber is important because it helps regulate blood sugar by reducing the amount of glucose absorbed from food. Your body works harder to digest foods that contain dietary fiber, and your intestines work more efficiently as well. Having adequate nutritional fiber can help reduce the risk for diabetes, heart disease, and obesity among other conditions. The Dietary Guidelines for Americans recommends 45–65 g. of protein per day, 30–45 g. of carbohydrate per day, and a moderate level of fat (20% or less) as part of a healthful diet for healthy people. The government also recommends 10–35 g. of fiber a day for healthy adults. The recommended level is higher for people with diabetes. A clinical trial showed that participants who received high-fiber cereal had lower blood sugar levels than participants who consumed a low-fiber cereal despite similar weight loss between groups. Participants who consumed the high-fiber cereal (13 g. per serving) had an average reduction in A1C of 0.28% points and post-breakfast blood sugar levels of 43 mg/dL; those who consumed the low-fiber cereal had average decreases of A1C of 0.03% points and post-breakfast blood sugar levels of 59 mg/dL.

Choose whole grains such as brown rice, whole wheat, oats, barley, and millet. Some other good sources include oat flour, cornmeal, flaxseed meal, wheat bran, and popcorn. Whole grains are high in fiber which will help you stay fuller for a longer period of time.

Chapter 5: Foods that Will Help the Infant to Get the Right Nutrients for Optimal Development

The foods that will help your baby to grow healthily.
The Foods that provide proper nourishment to the fetus, making it more difficult for diabetes and other complications in women.
Gestational Diabetes is when a woman's higher level of blood sugar than normal during her pregnancy causes complications of developing babies. Women are diagnosed with gestational diabetes 2 or more times in their pregnancy, before 20 weeks pregnant, or the end of 24 weeks pregnant. Gestational diabetes can cause some health risks to a baby. Those are macrosomia, neonatal hypoglycemia, hyperbilirubinemia, and shoulder dystocia.
Macrosomia is when babies have more than 8 lbs. at birth. Babies can get stressed during labor and delivery and have breathing problems after being born. A baby's shoulder can get stuck during delivery, causing an injury or even death. Babies with gestational diabetes can be born a month or more before their due date so that they would fit in the mother's pelvis for delivery. Babies born too soon, before 37 weeks of pregnancy, may have breathing problems that need special care in a NICU.
Neonatal hypoglycemia is when a newborn baby's blood sugar level is too low. Hypoglycemia can cause a baby's brain not to develop well. Babies with hypoglycemia need special care at a NICU.
Hyperbilirubinemia is when a newborn baby's blood has more bilirubin than normal. Too much bilirubin can hurt the brain and liver of newborn babies and can cause still birth for babies before 37 weeks of pregnancy.
So, the recommended food for the baby for development was the gestational diabetes diet that has the right balance of carbohydrates, protein, and fat.
Spreads for Gestational Diabetes (Gestational Diabetes Diet) in pregnancy, also known as bean sprouts, oilseeds, canola oil, avocado, are healthy for the mother and the baby. The recommended amount of gestational diabetes diet is about 75% of calories should be from whole grains. The remaining 25% should be consumed from fruits and vegetables, with leafy green vegetables being the only exception. The salt intake should be restricted to 6 g. per day or less (sodium chloride). Foods that are not recommended to pregnant women due to their high cholesterol and saturated fat content include eggs, salt substitutes, coconut oil, butter, margarine, meat products, and whole-fat dairy products.

For protein intake in gestational diabetes, the recommended amount is 0.25 g. per pound of body weight or 55 g. per day for a woman who weighs 150 lbs. The recommended amount of carbohydrate intake is also 0.25 g. per pound of body weight or 50 g. per day for a woman who weighs 150 lbs., which includes fiber intake recommended by the Institute of Medicine in 2000. There are many foods that contain carbohydrates, such as bread, cereal grains (oatmeal), rice, pasta, and beans.

The recommended fats for a gestational diabetes diet is 20% of total calories with most of the fats coming from oils, nuts and seeds. The essential fatty acids, which are omega-3s and omega-6s, are necessary for fetal growth and have been linked with healthier physical outcomes in children. Omega-3s are found in flaxseed (linseed), soybeans, walnuts, pumpkin seeds, and canola. Omega-6 is located in safflower oil, sunflower oil, peanuts, sesame seeds, and soybean oil.

Chapter 6: Foods that Raise Your Blood Sugar and Foods that Don't Raise Your Blood Sugar

What Do I Need to Eat If I Actually Have Gestational Diabetes?

A balanced weight-loss plan is key to correctly managing gestational diabetes. In other words, women with gestational diabetes should pay special attention to their carbohydrate, protein, and fat consumption. Eating often — as regularly as every two hours — also can help you to manipulate your blood sugar levels.

Carbohydrates

Your physician will assist you to decide precisely how many carbohydrates you should consume every day. They may additionally suggest that you see a registered dietician to help with meal plans. Healthy carbohydrate selections encompass:

- Complete grains
- Brown rice
- Beans, peas, lentils, and other legumes
- Starchy greens
- Low-sugar fruits

Protein

Pregnant ladies have to eat 2 to a few servings of protein each day. Good sources of protein encompass lean meats and rooster, fish, and tofu.

Fat

Healthy fats to incorporate into your eating regimen consist of unsalted nuts, seeds, olive oil, and avocado. Get extra guidelines right here on what to consume — and keep away from — when you have gestational diabetes.

What Complications Are Related to Gestational Diabetes?

If your gestational diabetes is under the weather organized, your blood sugar levels may also remain higher than they should be for the duration of your being pregnant. This can cause headaches and have an effect on the health of your toddler. For example, whilst your child is born, he or she may have:

- An excessive birth weight
- Breathing problems
- Low blood sugar
- Shoulder dystocia, which means their shoulders get caught inside the delivery canal at some point in labor

They can also be at risk of developing diabetes later in life. That's why it's so vital to take steps to manipulate your gestational diabetes by following your medical doctor's endorsed remedy plan.

What Is the Outlook for Gestational Diabetes?

Your blood sugar needs to return to ordinary after you give birth. But growing gestational diabetes increases your danger of type 2 diabetes later in existence. Ask your health practitioner how you could lower your risk of developing these situations and associated headaches.

Can Gestational Diabetes Be Prevented?

It's no longer feasible to save you gestational diabetes completely. However, adopting healthy habits can reduce your chances of growing the circumstance. If you're pregnant and feature one of the risk factors for gestational diabetes, attempt to devour a healthy weight-reduction plan and get an ordinary workout. Even light hobbies, including strolling, may be useful. If you're making plans to get pregnant within the near future, and also you're overweight, one of the best things you could do is work along with your medical doctor to lose weight. Even losing a small quantity of weight lets you lessen your risk of gestational diabetes.

Chapter 7: Meal Timing and Spacing

How Is Gestational Diabetes Controlled?

In general, gestational diabetes is controlled by the following: monitoring glucose levels, taking medications (if prescribed), proper weight gain for pregnancy, eating a good diet, getting regular exercise, and daily record keeping. Be sure to check with your healthcare provider for individualized information on each of these topics.
Gestational diabetes means that you are pregnant with a high blood sugar level. Food timing and spacing are of the utmost importance to manage gestational diabetes. There are also guidelines on the types of food to eat.

When to Eat?

Eat small meals throughout the day. A normal meal timing is to have 3 meals a day, but eat as many snacks as needed to prevent rising blood sugar levels.
If you get hungry between meals, eat slowly and finish your snack before you get up from the table. Do not drink soda, fruit juices, or alcohol while eating these snacks or at other times of the day. They help raise your blood sugar level. Instead, drink coffee or tea without sugar and eat food with protein in it.

Meal Spacing

Eat meals at fixed times and do not skip meals. This helps your body adjust its insulin production levels to your changing needs.
To keep blood sugar levels from going up after eating you may need to wait at times between eating the first meal of the day and the second or third food intake of the day. A general guideline is that there should be 2 hours from start to finish of each meal. If you make breakfast at 8 o'clock in the morning you can eat lunch at 10:30 am. After lunch, you can have small snacks until bedtime snack, which can be eaten 4 hours before going to bed (at least 2 hours before going to bed).

What Should I Eat?

A healthy diet is vital in any gestation. Proper carbohydrate intake is a key part of keeping glucose levels normal. Carbohydrate sources include grains, fruits, and vegetables. The carbs involved in these meal plans are slowly absorbed whole grains and lower glycemic index foods, which are less possible to raise blood glucose. It is helpful to eat smaller amounts of carbohydrates throughout the day rather than a large amount at one or two meals. This allows your body to metabolize the glucose produced from carbohydrates more efficiently. A small breakfast (that excludes fruit and fruit juice) is usually tolerated better than a larger breakfast. Many women find it helpful to include a bedtime snack in their meal plan. This booklet contains menus for 1800 calorie, 2000 calorie, and 2200 calorie diets.

Eat carbohydrates and protein with every meal. Avoid simple sugars from fruits and refined carbohydrates like cakes and pastries for snacks because they will increase your blood sugar level more than necessary.

Foods to Avoid

Avoid foods that contain high amounts of sugar or carbohydrates.
High carbohydrate foods include:

- Soft drinks (like soda), fruit juices, and fruit punches or punch mixed drinks.
- Candy bars, chocolate bars, and cakes.
- Sweets and baked goods like cookies, cakes, donuts, and pastries.
- Large portions of bread, rolls, and bagels with cream cheese or jelly. Bagels can have as many as seven g. of carbs each (one large plain bagel has 14 g.). Also, avoid white bread products (baguette, dinner roll) with the exception of sourdough bread which is OK in small amounts due to the naturally occurring yeast in them.

Chapter 8: Food Meal Plan

Day	Breakfast	Lunch	Snacks	Dinner
1	Berry Almond Smoothie	Baked Fennel and Garlic Sea Bass	Peanut Butter Sandwich Snacks	Apple Glazed Chicken with Spinach
2	Tropical Greek Yogurt Bowl	Cod & Green Bean Risotto	Baked Plantains	BBQ Ranch Wraps
3	Peanut Butter Power Oats	Mixed Pepper Stuffed River Trout	Strawberries and Cream Chocolate Cookie Sandwich	Baked Beans with Ground Beef
4	Blueberry Coconut Breakfast Cookies	Salad with Vinaigrette	Chocolate-Peppermint Thins	Baked Chicken Taquitos
5	Simple Grain-Free Biscuits	Herbed Chicken	Fall Harvest Salad	Beef and Vegetables in Peanut Sauce
6	Orange Muffins	Pesto Pork Chops	Two-Ingredient Ice Cream Cupcake Bites	Black Bean Queso Wraps
7	Crepe Cakes	Grilled Steak with Salsa	Lemon Blueberry Cheesecake Yogurt Bark	Buffalo Deviled Eggs

Chapter 9: Breakfast

1. Berry Almond Smoothie

Preparation time: 5 Minutes
Cooking time: 0 Minutes
Servings: 4
Ingredients

- 2 cups frozen berries of choice
- 1 cup plain low-fat Greek yogurt
- 1 cup unsweetened vanilla almond milk
- ½ cup natural almond butter

Directions

1. Put the berries, yogurt, almond milk, and almond butter into a blender, and blend until smooth. If the smoothie is too thick, add more almond milk to thin.

Nutrition

- Calories: 277
- Total Fat: 18 g.
- Protein: 13 g.
- Carbohydrates: 19 g.
- Sugars: 11 g.
- Fiber: 6 g.
- Sodium: 140 mg.

2. Tropical Greek Yogurt Bowl

Preparation time: 5 Minutes
Cooking time: 0 Minutes
Servings: 2
Ingredients
- 1 ½ cups plain low-fat Greek yogurt
- 2 kiwis, peeled and sliced
- 2 Tbsp. shredded unsweetened coconut flakes
- 2 Tbsp. halved walnuts
- 1 Tbsp. chia seeds
- 2 tsp. honey, divided (optional)

Directions
1. Divide the yogurt between 2 small bowls.
2. Top each serving of yogurt with half of the kiwi slices, coconut flakes, walnuts, chia seeds, and honey (if using).

Nutrition
- Calories: 260
- Total Fat: 9 g.
- Protein: 21 g.
- Carbohydrates: 23 g.
- Sugars: 14 g.
- Fiber: 6 g.
- Sodium: 83 mg.

3. Peanut Butter Power Oats

Preparation time: 5 Minutes
Cooking time: 5 Minutes
Servings: 2

Ingredients
- 1 ½ cups unsweetened vanilla almond milk
- ¾ cup rolled oats
- 1 Tbsp. chia seeds
- 2 Tbsp. natural peanut butter
- 2 Tbsp. walnut pieces, divided (optional)
- ¼ cup fresh berries, divided (optional)

Directions
1. In a small saucepan, bring the almond milk, oats, and chia seeds to a simmer.
2. Cover and cook, frequently stirring until all of the milk is absorbed and the chia seeds have gelled.
3. Add the peanut butter and stir until creamy.
4. Divide the oatmeal between two bowls. Top each serving with half of the walnuts and/or berries (if using).

Nutrition
- Calories: 261
- Total Fat: 14 g.
- Protein: 10 g.
- Carbohydrates: 27 g.
- Sugars: 1 g.
- Fiber: 7 g.
- Sodium: 131 mg.

4. Blueberry Coconut Breakfast Cookies

Preparation time: 10 Minutes
Cooking time: 15 Minutes
Servings: 4
Ingredients

- 4 Tbsp. unsalted butter, at room temperature
- 2 medium bananas
- 4 large eggs
- ½ cup unsweetened applesauce
- 1 tsp. vanilla extract
- ⅔ cup coconut flour
- ¼ tsp. salt
- 1 cup fresh or frozen blueberries

Directions

1. Preheat the oven to 375°F.
2. In a medium bowl, mash the butter and bananas together with a fork until combined. The bananas can be a little chunky.
3. Add the eggs, applesauce, and vanilla to the bananas and mix well.
4. Stir in the coconut flour and salt.
5. Gently fold in the blueberries.
6. Drop about 2 Tbsp.s of dough on a baking sheet for each cookie and flatten it a bit with the back of a spoon.
7. Bake for about 13 minutes or until firm to the touch.

Nutrition

- Calories: 305
- Total Fat: 18 g.
- Protein: 8 g.
- Carbohydrates: 28 g.
- Sugars: 15 g.
- Fiber: 7 g.
- Sodium: 222 mg.

5. Simple Grain-Free Biscuits

Preparation time: 10 Minutes
Cooking time: 15 Minutes
Servings: 4

Ingredients
- 2 Tbsp. unsalted butter
- Pinch salt
- ¼ cup plain low-fat Greek yogurt
- 1½ cups finely ground almond flour

Directions
1. Preheat the oven to 375°F.
2. In a medium bowl, microwave the butter just enough to soften, 15–20 seconds.
3. Add the salt and yogurt to the butter and mix well.
4. Add the almond flour and mix. The dough will be crumbly at first, so continue to stir and mash it with a fork until there are no lumps and the mixture comes together.
5. Drop ¼ cup of dough on a baking sheet for each biscuit. Using your clean hand, flatten each biscuit until it is 1 inch thick.
6. Bake for 13–15 minutes.

Nutrition
- Calories: 310
- Total Fat: 28 g.
- Protein: 10 g.
- Carbohydrates: 9 g.
- Sugars: 2 g.
- Fiber: 5 g.
- Sodium: 32 mg.

6. Orange Muffins

Preparation time: 15 Minutes
Cooking time: 15 Minutes
Servings: 9
Ingredients
- 2 ½ cups finely ground almond flour
- ¾ tsp. ground cinnamon
- ½ tsp. baking powder
- ½ tsp. ground cardamom
- ¼ tsp. salt
- 4 Tbsp. avocado or coconut oil
- 2 large eggs
- 1 medium orange, grated zest and juice
- 1 Tbsp. raw honey or 100% pure maple syrup
- ¼ tsp. vanilla extract

Directions
1. Preheat the oven to 375°F.
2. In a large bowl, whisk together the almond flour, cinnamon, baking powder, cardamom, and salt. Set aside.
3. In a medium bowl, whisk together the oil, eggs, zest, juice, honey, and vanilla. Add this mixture to the dry ingredients and stir until well combined.
4. In a nonstick muffin tin, fill each muffin cup until nearly full.
5. Bake for 15 minutes or until the top center is firm.

Nutrition
- Calories: 288
- Total Fat: 23.6 g.
- Protein: 8 g.
- Carbohydrates: 16 g.
- Sugars: 10 g.
- Fiber: 4 g.
- Sodium: 97 mg.

7. Crepe Cakes

Preparation time: 5 Minutes
Cooking time: 20 Minutes
Servings: 4

Ingredients
- Avocado oil cooking spray
- 4 oz. reduced-fat plain cream cheese, softened
- 2 medium bananas
- 4 large eggs
- ½ tsp. vanilla extract
- ⅛ tsp. salt

Directions
1. Heat a large skillet over low heat. Coat the cooking surface with cooking spray and allow the pan to heat for another 2 to 3 minutes.
2. Meanwhile, in a medium bowl, mash the cream cheese and bananas together with a fork until combined. The bananas can be a little chunky.
3. Add the eggs, vanilla, and salt, and mix well.
4. For each cake, drop 2 Tbsps. of the batter onto the warmed skillet and use the bottom of a large spoon or ladle to spread it thin. Let it cook for 7–9 minutes.
5. Flip the cake over and cook briefly for about 1 minute.

Nutrition
- Calories: 175
- Total Fat: 9 g.
- Protein: 9 g.
- Carbohydrates: 15 g.
- Sugars: 8 g.
- Fiber: 2 g.
- Sodium: 213 mg.

8. Coconut Pancakes

Preparation time: 5 Minutes
Cooking time: 20 Minutes
Servings: 4

Ingredients
- ½ cup coconut flour
- 1 tsp. baking powder
- ½ tsp. ground cinnamon
- ⅛ tsp. salt
- 8 large eggs
- ⅓ cup unsweetened almond milk
- 2 Tbsp. avocado or coconut oil
- 1 tsp. vanilla extract

Directions
1. Heat a large skillet over medium-low heat.
2. In a large bowl, whisk together the flour, baking powder, cinnamon, and salt. Set aside.
3. In a medium bowl, whisk together the eggs, almond milk, oil, and vanilla. Pour the wet mixture into the dry ingredients and stir until combined.
4. Pour ⅓ cup of the batter onto the skillet for each pancake. Cook until bubbles appear on the surface of the pancake, about 7 minutes, then flip and cook for 1 minute more.

Nutrition
- Calories: 270
- Total Fat: 18 g.
- Protein: 14 g.
- Carbohydrates: 10 g.
- Sugars: 2 g.
- Fiber: 5 g.
- Sodium: 325 mg.

9. Loaded Avocado

Preparation time: 5 Minutes
Cooking time: 5 Minutes
Servings: 4

Ingredients
- Avocado oil cooking spray
- 8 large eggs
- 2 avocados
- ¼ cup roasted red pepper spread
- Fresh cilantro leaves, for garnish
- Lime wedges, for garnish

Directions
1. Heat a large skillet over medium heat. When hot, coat the cooking surface with cooking spray and cook the eggs to your liking.
2. Meanwhile, cut the avocados in half lengthwise and remove the pits. Top each avocado half with 1 Tbsp. of the red pepper spread.
3. For each portion, serve 2 eggs alongside 1 avocado half and garnish with cilantro and a lime wedge.

Nutrition
- Calories: 250
- Total Fat: 20 g.
- Protein: 16 g.
- Carbohydrates: 18 g.
- Sugars: 2 g.
- Fiber: 5 g.
- Sodium: 325 mg.

10. Breakfast Tacos

Preparation time: 5 Minutes
Cooking time: 10 Minutes
Servings: 4
Ingredients
For the taco filling:
- Avocado oil cooking spray
- 1 medium green bell pepper, chopped
- 8 large eggs
- ¼ cup shredded sharp Cheddar cheese
- 4 (6-inch) whole-wheat tortillas
- 1 cup fresh spinach leaves
- ½ cup Pico de Gallo
- Scallions, chopped, for garnish (optional)
- Avocado slices, for garnish (optional)

For the Pico de Gallo:
- 1 tomato, diced
- ½ large white onion, diced
- 2 Tbsp.s chopped fresh cilantro
- ½ jalapeño pepper, stemmed, seeded, and diced
- 1 Tbsp. freshly squeezed lime juice
- ⅛ tsp. salt

Directions
To make the taco filling:
1. Heat a medium skillet over medium-low heat. When hot, coat the cooking surface with cooking spray and put the pepper in the skillet. Cook for 4 minutes.
2. Meanwhile, whisk the eggs in a medium bowl, then add the cheese and whisk to combine. Pour the eggs and cheese into the skillet with the green peppers and scramble until the eggs are fully cooked, about 5 minutes.
3. Microwave the tortillas very briefly, about 8 seconds.

4. For each serving top a tortilla with one-quarter of the spinach, eggs, and Pico de Gallo. Garnish with scallions and avocado slices (if using).

To make the Pico de Gallo:
1. In a medium bowl, combine the tomato, onion, cilantro, pepper, lime juice, and salt. Mix well and serve.

Nutrition
- Calories: 276
- Total Fat: 12 g.
- Protein: 16 g.
- Carbohydrates: 28 g.
- Sugars: 8 g.
- Fiber: 3 g.
- Sodium: 562 mg.

11. Huevos Rancheros Remix

Preparation time: 5 Minutes
Cooking time: 10 Minutes
Servings: 4

Ingredients

- 1 cup low-sodium black beans, drained and rinsed
- Avocado oil cooking spray
- ½ cup jarred salsa Verde
- 8 large eggs
- 1 cup packaged or fresh Pico de Gallo
- 4 lime wedges

Directions

1. Pour the black beans and salsa Verde into a small saucepan over low heat and cover. Cook until the beans are heated through, about 10 minutes.
2. Meanwhile, heat a small skillet over medium-low heat. When hot, coat the cooking surface with cooking spray and fry or scramble the eggs to your liking.
3. For each portion, top 2 eggs with one-quarter of the black beans and Pico de Gallo. Finish each portion with a squeeze of lime.

Nutrition

- Calories: 210
- Total Fat: 9.4 g.
- Protein: 15 g.
- Carbohydrates: 18 g.
- Sugars: 4 g.
- Fiber: 5 g.
- Sodium: 439 mg.

12. Brussels Sprouts and Egg Scramble

Preparation time: 5 Minutes
Cooking time: 10 Minutes
Servings: 4

Ingredients

- Avocado oil cooking spray
- 4 slices low-sodium turkey bacon
- 20 Brussels sprouts, halved lengthwise
- 8 large eggs
- ¼ cup crumbled feta, for garnish

Directions

1. Heat a large skillet over medium heat. When hot, coat the cooking surface with cooking spray and cook the bacon to your liking.
2. Carefully remove the bacon from the pan and set it on a plate lined with a paper towel to drain and cool.
3. Place the Brussels sprouts in the skillet cut-side down and cook for 3 minutes.
4. Reduce the heat to medium-low. Flip the Brussels sprouts, move them to one side of the skillet, and cover. Cook for another 3 minutes.
5. Uncover. Cook the eggs to over-medium alongside the Brussels sprouts or to your liking.
6. Crumble the bacon once it has cooled.
7. Divide the Brussels sprouts into 4 portions and top each portion with one-quarter of the crumbled bacon and 2 eggs. Add 1 Tbsp. of feta to each portion.

Nutrition

- Calories: 253
- Total Fat: 15 g.
- Protein: 21 g.
- Carbohydrates: 10 g.
- Sugars: 4 g.
- Fiber: 4 g.
- Sodium: 343 mg.

13. Sausage, Sweet Potato, and Kale Hash

Preparation time: 10 Minutes
Cooking time: 15 Minutes
Servings: 4
Ingredients
- Avocado oil cooking spray
- 1 ⅓ cups peeled and diced sweet potatoes
- 8 cups roughly chopped kale, stemmed and loosely packed (about 2 bunches)
- 4 links chicken or turkey breakfast sausage
- 4 large eggs
- 4 lemon wedges

Directions
1. Heat a large skillet over medium heat. When hot, coat the cooking surface with cooking spray. Cook the sweet potatoes for 4 minutes, stirring once halfway through.
2. Reduce the heat to medium-low and move the potatoes to one side of the skillet. Arrange the kale and sausage in a single layer. Cover and cook for 3 minutes.
3. Stir the vegetables and sausage together, then push them to one side of the skillet to create space for the eggs. Add the eggs and cook them to your liking. Cover the skillet and cook for 3 minutes.
4. Divide the sausage and vegetables into four equal portions and top with an egg and a squeeze of lemon.

Nutrition
- Calories: 234
- Total Fat: 8 g.
- Protein: 12 g.
- Carbohydrates: 32 g.
- Sugars: 6 g.
- Fiber: 5 g.
- Sodium: 270 mg.

14. Maple Sausage Frittata

Preparation time: 10 Minutes
Cooking time: 15 Minutes
Servings: 4

Ingredients

- Avocado oil cooking spray
- 1 cup roughly chopped portobello mushrooms
- 1 medium green bell pepper, diced
- 1 medium red bell pepper, diced
- 8 large eggs
- ¾ cup half-and-half
- ¼ cup unsweetened almond milk
- 6 links maple-flavored chicken or turkey breakfast sausage, cut into ¼-inch pieces

Directions

1. Preheat the oven to 375°F.
2. Heat a large, oven-safe skillet over medium-low heat. When hot, coat the cooking surface with cooking spray.
3. Heat the mushrooms, green bell pepper, and red bell pepper in the skillet. Cook for 5 minutes.
4. Meanwhile, in a medium bowl, whisk the eggs, half-and-half, and almond milk.
5. Add the sausage to the skillet and cook for 2 minutes.
6. Pour the egg mixture into the skillet, then transfer the skillet from the stove to the oven and bake for 15 minutes or until the middle is firm and spongy.

Nutrition

- Calories: 280
- Total Fat: 17 g.
- Protein: 21 g.
- Carbohydrates: 10 g.
- Sugars: 7 g.
- Fiber: 2 g.
- Sodium: 446 mg.

15. Coconut-Berry Sunrise Smoothie

Preparation time: 5 Minutes
Cooking time: 0 Minutes
Servings: 2
Ingredients

- ½ cup mixed berries (blueberries, strawberries, blackberries)
- 1 Tbsp. ground flaxseed
- 2 Tbsp. unsweetened coconut flakes
- ½ cup unsweetened plain coconut milk
- ½ cup leafy greens (kale, spinach)
- ¼ cup unsweetened vanilla nonfat yogurt
- ½ cup ice

Directions

1. In a blender jar, combine the berries, flaxseed, coconut flakes, coconut milk, greens, yogurt, and ice.
2. Process until smooth. Serve.

Nutrition

- Calories: 181
- Total Fat: 15 g.
- Protein: 6 g.
- Carbohydrates: 8 g.
- Sugars: 3 g.
- Fiber: 4 g.
- Sodium: 24 mg.

16. Avocado and Goat Cheese Toast

Preparation time: 5 Minutes
Cooking time: 5 Minutes
Servings: 2
Ingredients
- 2 slices whole-wheat thin-sliced bread (I love Ezekiel sprouted bread and Dave's Killer Bread)
- ½ avocado
- 2 Tbsp. crumbled goat cheese
- Salt

Directions
1. In a toaster or broiler, toast the bread until browned.
2. Remove the flesh from the avocado. In a medium bowl, use a fork to mash the avocado flesh. Spread it onto the toast.
3. Sprinkle with the goat cheese and season lightly with salt.
4. Add any toppings and serve.

Nutrition
- Calories: 137
- Total Fat: 6 g.
- Protein: 5 g.
- Carbohydrates: 18 g.
- Sugars: 0 g.
- Fiber: 5 g.
- Sodium: 195 mg.

17. Oat and Walnut Granola

Preparation time: 10 Minutes
Cooking time: 30 Minutes
Servings: 16

Ingredients

- 4 cups rolled oats
- 1 cup walnut pieces
- ½ cup pepitas
- ¼ tsp. salt
- 1 tsp. ground cinnamon
- 1 tsp. ground ginger
- ½ cup coconut oil, melted
- ½ cup unsweetened applesauce
- 1 tsp. vanilla extract
- ½ cup dried cherries

Directions

1. Preheat the oven to 350°F. Line a baking sheet with parchment paper.
2. In a large bowl, toss the oats, walnuts, pepitas, salt, cinnamon, and ginger.
3. In a large measuring cup, combine the coconut oil, applesauce, and vanilla. Pour over the dry mixture and mix well
4. Transfer the mixture to the prepared baking sheet. Cook for 30 minutes, stirring about halfway through. Remove from the oven and let the granola sit undisturbed until completely cool. Break the granola into pieces, and stir in the dried cherries.
5. Transfer to an airtight container, and store at room temperature for up to 2 weeks.

Nutrition

- Calories: 224
- Total Fat: 15 g.
- Protein: 5 g.
- Carbohydrates: 20 g. - Sugars: 5 g. - Fiber: 3 g.
- Sodium: 30 mg.

18. Chocolate-Zucchini Muffins

Preparation time: 15 Minutes - **Cooking time:** 20 Minutes
Servings: 12 - **Ingredients**

- 1½ cups grated zucchini
- 1½ cups rolled oats; 1 tsp. ground cinnamon
- 2 tsp. baking powder
- ¼ tsp. salt; 1 large egg
- 1 tsp. vanilla extract
- ¼ cup coconut oil, melted
- ½ cup unsweetened applesauce; ¼ cup honey
- ¼ cup dark chocolate chips

Directions

1. Preheat the oven to 350°F. Grease the cups of a 12-cup muffin tin or line with paper baking liners. Set aside.
2. Place the zucchini in a colander over the sink to drain.
3. In a blender jar, process the oats until they resemble flour. Transfer to a medium mixing bowl and add the cinnamon, baking powder, and salt. Mix well.
4. In another large mixing bowl, combine the egg, vanilla, coconut oil, applesauce, and honey. Stir to combine.
5. Press the zucchini into the colander, draining any liquids, and add to the wet mixture.
6. Stir the dry mixture into the wet mixture and mix until no dry spots remain. Fold in the chocolate chips.
7. Transfer the batter to the muffin tin, filling each cup a little over halfway. Cook for 16 to 18 minutes until the muffins are lightly browned and a toothpick inserted in the center comes out clean.
8. Store in an airtight container, refrigerated, for up to 5 days.

Nutrition

- Calories: 121 - Total Fat: 7 g.
- Protein: 2 g. - Carbohydrates: 16 g. - Sugars: 7 g. - Fiber: 2 g. - Sodium: 106 mg.

19. Gluten-Free Carrot and Oat Pancakes

Preparation time: 10 Minutes
Cooking time: 20 Minutes
Servings: 4
Ingredients

- 1 cup rolled oats
- 1 cup shredded carrots
- 1 cup low-fat cottage cheese
- 2 eggs
- ½ cup unsweetened plain almond milk
- 1 tsp. baking powder
- ½ tsp. ground cinnamon
- 2 Tbsp. ground flaxseed
- ¼ cup plain nonfat Greek yogurt
- 1 Tbsp. pure maple syrup
- 2 tsp. canola oil, divided

Directions

1. In a blender jar, process the oats until they resemble flour. Add the carrots, cottage cheese, eggs, almond milk, baking powder, cinnamon, and flaxseed to the jar. Process until smooth.
2. In a small bowl, combine the yogurt and maple syrup, and stir well. Set aside.
3. In a large skillet, heat 1 tsp. of oil over medium heat. Using a measuring cup, add ¼ cup of batter per pancake to the skillet. Cook for 1–2 minutes until bubbles form on the surface, then flip the pancakes. Cook for another minute until the pancakes are browned and cooked through. Repeat with the remaining 1 tsp. of oil and remaining batter.
4. Serve warm topped with maple yogurt.

Nutrition

- Calories: 226 - Total Fat: 8 g. - Protein: 15 g. - Carbohydrates: 24 g.
- Sugars: 7 g.
- Fiber: 4 g.
- Sodium: 403 mg.

20. Breakfast Egg Bites

Preparation time: 10 Minutes
Cooking time: 25 Minutes
Servings: 8

Ingredients

- Nonstick cooking spray
- 6 eggs, beaten
- ¼ cup unsweetened plain almond milk
- 1 red bell pepper, diced
- 1 cup chopped spinach
- ¼ cup crumbled goat cheese
- ½ cup sliced brown mushrooms
- ¼ cup sliced sun-dried tomatoes
- Salt
- Freshly ground black pepper

Directions

1. Preheat the oven to 350°F. Spray 8 muffin cups of a 12-cup muffin tin with nonstick cooking spray. Set aside.
2. In a large mixing bowl, combine the eggs, almond milk, bell pepper, spinach, goat cheese, mushrooms, and tomatoes. Season with salt and pepper.
3. Fill the prepared muffin cups three-fourths full with the egg mixture. Bake for 20–25 minutes until the eggs are set. Let cool slightly and remove the egg bites from the muffin tin.
4. Serve warm, or store in an airtight container in the refrigerator for up to 5 days, or in the freezer for up to 1 month.

Nutrition

- Calories: 67 - Total Fat: 4 g. - Protein: 6 g. - Carbohydrates: 3 g.
- Sugars: 2 g.
- Fiber: 1 g.
- Sodium: 127 mg.

21. Spinach, Artichoke, and Goat Cheese Breakfast Bake

Preparation time: 10 Minutes
Cooking time: 35 Minutes
Servings: 8

Ingredients

- 1 (10-oz.) package frozen spinach, thawed and drained
- 1 (14-oz.) can artichoke hearts, drained
- ¼ cup finely chopped red bell pepper
- 2 garlic cloves, minced
- 8 eggs, lightly beaten
- ¼ cup unsweetened plain almond milk
- ½ tsp. salt
- ½ tsp. freshly ground black pepper
- ½ cup crumbled goat cheese

Directions

1. Preheat the oven to 375°F. Spray an 8-by-8-inch baking dish with nonstick cooking spray.
2. In a large mixing bowl, combine the spinach, artichoke hearts, bell pepper, garlic, eggs, almond milk, salt, and pepper. Stir well to combine.
3. Transfer the mixture to the baking dish. Sprinkle with the goat cheese.
4. Bake for 35 minutes until the eggs are set. Serve warm.

Nutrition

- Calories: 104
- Total Fat: 5 g.
- Protein: 9 g.
- Carbohydrates: 6 g.
- Sugars: 1 g.
- Fiber: 2 g.
- Sodium: 488 mg.

22. Crispy Breakfast Pita With Egg and Canadian Bacon

Preparation time: 5 Minutes
Cooking time: 15 Minutes
Servings: 2
Ingredients

- 1 (6-inch) whole-grain pita bread
- 3 tsp. extra-virgin olive oil, divided
- 2 eggs
- 2 Canadian bacon slices
- ½ lemon, juiced
- 1 cup microgreens
- 2 Tbsp. crumbled goat cheese
- Freshly ground black pepper

Directions

1. Heat a large skillet over medium heat. Cut the pita bread in half and brush each side of both halves with ¼ tsp. of olive oil (using a total of 1 tsp. oil). Cook for 2–3 minutes on each side, then remove from the skillet.
2. In the same skillet, heat 1 tsp. of oil over medium heat. Crack the eggs into the skillet and cook until the eggs are set, 2–3 minutes. Remove from the skillet.
3. In the same skillet, cook the Canadian bacon for 3–5 minutes, flipping once.
4. In a large bowl, whisk together the remaining 1 tsp. of oil and lemon juice. Add the microgreens and toss to combine.
5. Top each pita half with half of the microgreens, 1 piece of bacon, 1 egg, and 1 Tbsp. of goat cheese. Season with pepper and serve.

Nutrition

- Calories: 250 - Total Fat: 14 g. - Protein: 13 g.
- Carbohydrates: 20 g.
- Sugars: 1 g.
- Fiber: 3 g.
- Sodium: 398 mg.

23. Brussels Sprout Hash and Eggs

Preparation time: 15 Minutes
Cooking time: 15 Minutes
Servings: 4

Ingredients
- 3 tsp. extra-virgin olive oil, divided
- 1 lb. Brussels sprouts, sliced
- 2 garlic cloves, thinly sliced
- ¼ tsp. salt
- 1 lemon, Juice
- 4 eggs

Directions
1. In a large skillet, heat 1½ tsp. of oil over medium heat. Add the Brussels sprouts and toss. Cook, stirring regularly, for 6–8 minutes until browned and softened. Add the garlic and continue to cook until fragrant, about 1 minute. Season with salt and lemon juice. Transfer to a serving dish.
2. In the same pan, heat the remaining 1½ tsp.s of oil over medium-high heat. Crack the eggs into the pan. Fry for 2–4 minutes, flip and continue cooking to desired doneness. Serve over the bed of hash.

Nutrition
- Calories: 158
- Total Fat: 9 g.
- Protein: 10 g.
- Carbohydrates: 12 g.
- Sugars: 4 g.
- Fiber: 4 g.
- Sodium: 234 mg.

Chapter 10: Lunch

24. Shrimp Paella

Preparation time: 5 Minutes
Cooking time: 10 Minutes
Servings: 2
Ingredients

- 1 cup cooked brown rice
- 1 chopped red onion
- 1 tsp. paprika
- 1 chopped garlic clove
- 1 Tbsp. olive oil
- 6 oz. frozen cooked shrimp
- 1 deseeded and sliced chili pepper
- 1 Tbsp. oregano

Directions

1. Warm the olive oil in a pan on medium-high heat.
2. Add the onion and garlic, and sauté for 2–3 minutes until soft.
3. Now add the shrimp and sauté for a further 5 minutes or until hot through.
4. Then add the herbs, spices, chili and rice with ½ cup boiling water.
5. Stir until everything is warm and the water has been absorbed.
6. Plate up and serve.

Nutrition

- Calories: 221
- Protein: 17 g.
- Carbs: 31 g.
- Fat: 8 g.
- Sodium (Na): 235 mg.
- Potassium (K): 176 mg.
- Phosphorus: 189 mg.

25. Salmon and Pesto Salad

Preparation time: 5 Minutes - **Cooking time:** 15 Minutes
Servings: 2 - **Ingredients**
For the pesto:
- 1 minced garlic clove
- ½ cup fresh arugula
- ¼ cup extra virgin olive oil
- ½ cup fresh basil
- 1 tsp. black pepper

For the salmon:
- 4 oz. skinless salmon fillet
- 1 Tbsp. coconut oil

For the salad:
- ½ juiced lemon; 2 sliced radishes
- ½ cup iceberg lettuce
- 1 tsp. black pepper

Directions

1. Prepare the pesto by blending all the pesto ingredients in a food processor or grinding with a pestle and mortar. Set aside.
2. Put a skillet over the stove on medium-high heat and melt the coconut oil.
3. Add the salmon to the pan.
4. Cook for 7–8 minutes and turn over.
5. Cook for an additional 3–4 minutes or up until cooked through.
6. Remove fillets from the skillet and allow to rest.
7. Mix the lettuce and radishes and squeeze over the juice of ½ lemon.
8. Flake the salmon with a fork and mix through the salad.
9. Toss to coat and sprinkle with a little black pepper to serve.

Nutrition

- Calories: 221- Protein: 13 g. - Carbs: 1 g. - Fat: 34 g. - Sodium: (Na): 80 mg.
- Potassium (K): 119 mg. - Phosphorus: 158 mg.

26. Baked Fennel and Garlic Sea Bass

Preparation time: 5 Minutes
Cooking time: 15 Minutes
Servings: 2
Ingredients

- 1 lemon
- ½ sliced fennel bulb
- 6 oz. sea bass fillets
- 1 tsp. black pepper
- 2 garlic cloves

Directions

1. Preheat the oven to 375°F/Gas Spot 5.
2. Sprinkle black pepper over the Sea Bass.
3. Slice the fennel bulb and garlic cloves.
4. Add 1 salmon fillet and half the fennel and garlic to 1 sheet of baking paper or tin foil.
5. Squeeze in ½ lemon juices.
6. Repeat for the other fillet.
7. Fold and put in the oven for 12–15 minutes or until fish is thoroughly cooked through.
8. Meanwhile, add boiling water to your couscous, cover, and allow to steam.
9. Serve with your choice of rice or salad.

Nutrition

- Calories: 221
- Protein: 14 g.
- Carbs: 3 g.
- Fat: 2 g.
- Sodium (Na): 119 mg.
- Potassium (K): 398 mg.
- Phosphorus: 149 mg.

27. Lemon, Garlic, and Cilantro Tuna and Rice

Preparation time: 5 Minutes
Cooking time: 0 Minutes
Servings: 2

Ingredients

- ½ cup arugula
- 1 Tbsp. extra-virgin olive oil
- 1 cup cooked rice
- 1 tsp. black pepper
- ¼ finely diced red onion
- 1 lemon, juice
- 3 oz. canned tuna
- 2 Tbsp. chopped fresh cilantro

Directions

1. Mix the olive oil, pepper, cilantro, and red onion in a bowl.
2. Stir in the tuna, cover, and leave in the fridge for as long as possible. Serve immediately.
3. When ready to eat, serve up with the cooked rice and arugula!

Nutrition

- Calories: 221
- Protein: 11 g.
- Carbs: 26 g.
- Fat: 7 g.
- Sodium (Na): 143 mg.
- Potassium (K): 197 mg.
- Phosphorus: 182 mg.

28. Cod and Green Bean Risotto

Preparation time: 4 Minutes - **Cooking time:** 40 Minutes
Servings: 2 - **Ingredients**

- ½ cup arugula
- 1 finely diced white onion
- 4 oz. cod fillet
- 1 cup white rice
- 2 lemon wedges
- 1 cup boiling water
- ¼ tsp. black pepper
- 1 cup low sodium chicken broth
- 1 Tbsp. extra-virgin olive oil
- ½ cup green beans

Directions

1. Heat the oil in a large pan on standard heat.
2. Sauté the chopped onion for 5 minutes until soft before adding in the rice and stirring for 1–2 minutes.
3. Combine the broth with boiling water.
4. Add half of the liquid to the pan and stir slowly.
5. Slowly add the rest of the liquid while continuously stirring for up to 20–30 minutes.
6. Stir in the green beans to the risotto.
7. Place the fish on top of the rice, cover, and steam for 10 minutes.
8. Ensure the water does not dry out and keep topping up until the rice is cooked thoroughly.
9. Use your fork to break up the fish fillets and stir them into the rice.
10. Sprinkle with freshly ground pepper to serve and a squeeze of fresh lemon.
11. Garnish with lemon wedges and serve with the arugula.

Nutrition

- Calories: 221-Protein: 12 g.-Carbs: 29 g.-Fat: 8 g.-Sodium (Na): 398 mg. Potassium (K): 347 mg.
- Phosphorus: 241 mg.

29. Mixed Pepper Stuffed River Trout

Preparation time: 5 Minutes
Cooking time: 20 Minutes
Servings: 4
Ingredients
- 1 whole river trout
- 1 tsp. thyme
- ¼ diced yellow pepper
- 1 cup baby spinach leaves
- ¼ diced green pepper
- 1 juiced lime
- ¼ diced red pepper
- 1 tsp. oregano
- 1 tsp. extra-virgin olive oil
- 1 tsp. black pepper

Directions
1. Preheat the broiler/grill on high heat.
2. Lightly oil a baking tray.
3. Mix all of the fixings apart from the trout and lime.
4. Slice the trout lengthways (there should be an opening here from where it was gutted) and stuff the mixed ingredients inside.
5. Squeeze the lime juice over the fish and then place the lime wedges on the tray.
6. Place under the broiler on the baking tray and broil for 15–20 minutes or until fish is thoroughly cooked through and flakes easily.
7. Enjoy alone or with a side helping of rice or salad.

Nutrition
- Calories: 290
- Protein: 15 g.
- Carbs: 0 g.
- Fat: 7 g.- Sodium (Na): 43 mg.-Potassium (K): 315 mg.-Phosphorus: 189 mg.

30. Haddock and Buttered Leeks

Preparation time: 5 Minutes
Cooking time: 15 Minutes
Servings: 2
Ingredients

- 1 Tbsp. unsalted butter
- 1 sliced leek
- ¼ tsp. black pepper
- 2 tsp. chopped parsley
- 6 oz. haddock fillets
- ½ juiced lemon

Directions

1. Preheat the oven to 375°F/Gas Mark 5.
2. Add the haddock fillets to baking or parchment paper and sprinkle with the black pepper.
3. Squeeze over the lemon juice and wrap it into a parcel.
4. Bake the parcel on a baking tray for 10–15 minutes or until the fish is thoroughly cooked through.
5. Meanwhile, heat the butter over medium-low heat in a small pan.
6. Add the leeks and parsley, and sauté for 5–7 minutes until soft.
7. Serve the haddock fillets on a bed of buttered leeks, and enjoy!

Nutrition

- Calories: 124
- Protein: 15 g.
- Carbs: 0 g.
- Fat: 7 g.
- Sodium (Na): 161 mg.
- Potassium (K): 251 mg.
- Phosphorus: 220 mg.

31. Thai Spiced Halibut

Preparation time: 5 Minutes
Cooking time: 20 Minutes
Servings: 2

Ingredients
- 2 Tbsp. coconut oil
- 1 cup white rice
- ¼ tsp. black pepper
- ½ diced red chili
- 1 Tbsp. fresh basil
- 2 pressed garlic cloves
- 4 oz. halibut fillet
- 1 halved lime
- 2 sliced green onions
- 1 lime leaf

Directions
1. Preheat oven to 400°F/Gas Mark 5.
2. Add half of the ingredients into baking paper and fold into a parcel.
3. Repeat for your second parcel.
4. Cook in the oven for 15–20 minutes or until fish is thoroughly cooked through.
5. Serve with cooked rice.

Nutrition
- Calories: 311
- Protein: 16 g.
- Carbs: 17 g.
- Fat: 15 g.
- Sodium (Na): 31 mg.
- Potassium (K): 418 mg.
- Phosphorus: 257 mg.

32. Homemade Tuna Niçoise

Preparation time: 5 Minutes
Cooking time: 10 Minutes
Servings: 2
Ingredients
- 1 egg
- ½ cup green beans
- ¼ sliced cucumber
- 1 lemon, juiced
- 1 tsp. black pepper
- ¼ sliced red onion
- 1 Tbsp. olive oil
- 1 Tbsp. capers
- 4 oz. drained canned tuna
- 4 leaves iceberg lettuce
- 1 tsp. chopped fresh cilantro

Directions
1. Prepare the salad by washing and slicing the lettuce, cucumber, and onion.
2. Add to a salad bowl.
3. Mix 1 tbsp oil with lemon juice, cilantro, and capers for a salad dressing. Set aside.
4. Boil a pan of water on high heat, then lower to simmer and add the egg for 6 minutes. (Steam the green beans over the same pan in a steamer/colander for 6 minutes.)
5. Remove the egg and rinse under cold water.
6. Peel before slicing in half.
7. Mix the tuna, salad and dressing together in a salad bowl.
8. Toss to coat.
9. Top with the egg and serve with a sprinkle of black pepper.

Nutrition
- Calories: 199-Protein: 19 g.-Carbs: 7 g.
- Fat: 8 g.-Sodium (Na): 466 mg.-Potassium (K): 251 mg.-Phosphorus: 211 mg.

33. Monkfish Curry

Preparation time: 5 Minutes
Cooking time: 20 Minutes
Servings: 2
Ingredients
- 1 garlic clove
- 3 finely chopped green onions
- 1 tsp. grated ginger
- 1 cup 1 water.
- 2 tsp. chopped fresh basil
- 1 cup cooked rice noodles
- 1 Tbsp. coconut oil
- ½ sliced red chili
- 4 oz. Monkfish fillet
- ½ finely sliced stick lemon-grass
- 2 Tbsp. chopped shallots

Directions
1. Slice the monkfish into bite-size pieces.
2. By means of a pestle, also mortar or food processor, crush the basil, garlic, ginger, chili, and lemon-grass to form a paste.
3. Heat the oil in a pan over medium-high heat and add the shallots.
4. Now add the water to the pan and bring to a boil.
5. Add the Monkfish, lower the heat, and cover to simmer for 10 minutes or until cooked through.
6. Enjoy with rice noodles and scatter with green onions to serve.

Nutrition
- Calories: 249-Protein: 12 g.-Carbs: 30 g.-Fat: 10 g.
- Sodium (Na): 32 mg.
- Potassium (K): 398 mg.
- Phosphorus: 190 mg.

34. Salad With Vinaigrette

Preparation time: 25 Minutes
Cooking time: 0 Minutes
Servings: 4
Ingredients
For the vinaigrette:
- ½ cup olive oil
- 4 Tbsps. balsamic vinegar
- 2 Tbsps. chopped fresh oregano
- Pinch red pepper flakes
- Ground black pepper

For the salad:
- 4 cups shredded green leaf lettuce
- 1 carrot, shredded
- ¾ cup fresh green beans, cut into 1-inch pieces
- 3 large radishes, sliced thin

Directions
To make the vinaigrette:
1. Put the vinaigrette ingredients in a bowl and whisk.
2. In a bowl, make the salad; pitch together with the carrot, lettuce, green beans, and radishes.
3. Add the vinaigrette to the vegetables and toss to coat.
4. Arrange the salad on plates and serve.

Nutrition
- Calories: 273
- Fat: 27 g.
- Carb: 7 g.
- Phosphorus: 30 mg.
- Potassium: 197 mg.
- Sodium: 27 mg.
- Protein: 1 g.

35. Salad With Lemon Dressing

Preparation time: 10 Minutes
Cooking time: 0 Minutes
Servings: 4

Ingredients

- ¼ cup heavy cream
- ¼ cup freshly squeezed lemon juice
- 2 Tbsp. granulated sugar
- 2 Tbsp. chopped fresh dill
- 2 Tbsps. finely chopped scallion, green part only
- ¼ tsp. ground black pepper
- 1 English cucumber, sliced thin
- 2 cups shredded green cabbage

Directions

1. In a small bowl, mix the lemon juice, cream, sugar, dill, scallion, and pepper until well blended.
2. In a large bowl, toss together the cucumber and cabbage.
3. Place the salad in the refrigerator and chill for 1 hour.
4. Stir before serving.

Nutrition

- Calories: 99
- Fat: 6 g.
- Carb: 13 g.
- Phosphorus: 38 mg.
- Potassium: 200 mg.
- Sodium: 14 mg.
- Protein: 2 g.

36. Shrimp With Salsa

Preparation time: 15 Minutes
Cooking time: 10 Minutes
Servings: 4

Ingredients

- 2 Tbsp. olive oil
- 6 oz. large shrimp, peeled and deveined, tails left on
- 1 tsp. minced garlic
- ½ cup chopped English cucumber
- ½ cup chopped mango
- Zest of 1 lime
- Juice of 1 lime
- Ground black pepper
- Lime wedges for garnish

Directions

1. Soak 4 wooden skewers in water for 30 minutes.
2. Preheat the barbecue to medium heat.
3. In a bowl, toss together the olive oil, shrimp, and garlic.
4. Thread the shrimp onto the skewers, about four shrimp per skewer.
5. In a bowl, stir together the mango, cucumber, lime zest, and lime juice, and season the salsa lightly with pepper. Set aside.
6. Grill the shrimp for 10 minutes, turning once or until the shrimp is opaque and cooked through.
7. Season the shrimp lightly with pepper.
8. Serve the shrimp on the cucumber salsa with lime wedges on the side.

Nutrition

- Calories: 120 -Fat: 8 g. -Carb: 4 g.
- Phosphorus: 91 mg. - Potassium: 129 mg.
- Sodium: 60 mg.
- Protein: 9 g.

37. Cauliflower Soup

Preparation time: 20 Minutes
Cooking time: 30 Minutes
Servings: 6
Ingredients
- 1 tsp. unsalted butter
- 1 small sweet onion, chopped
- 2 tsp. minced garlic
- 1 small head cauliflower, cut into small florets
- 2 tsp. curry powder
- Water to cover the cauliflower
- ½ cup light sour cream
- 3 Tbsp. chopped fresh cilantro

Directions
1. In a large saucepan, heat the butter over medium-high heat and sauté the onion-garlic for about 3 minutes or until softened.
2. Add the cauliflower, water, and curry powder.
3. Bring the solution to a boil, then reduce the heat to low and simmer for 20 minutes or until the cauliflower is tender.
4. Puree the soup until creamy and smooth with a hand mixer.
5. Transfer the soup back into a pan and stir in the sour cream and cilantro.
6. Heat the soup on medium heat for 5 minutes or until warmed through.

Nutrition
- Calories: 33
- Fat: 2 g.
- Carb: 4 g.
- Phosphorus: 30 mg.
- Potassium: 167 mg.
- Sodium: 22 mg.
- Protein: 1 g.

38. Cabbage Stew

Preparation time: 20 Minutes - **Cooking time:** 35 Minutes
Servings: 6 - **Ingredients**
- 1 tsp. unsalted butter
- ½ large sweet onion, chopped
- 1 tsp. minced garlic
- 6 cups shredded green cabbage
- 3 celery stalks, chopped with leafy tops
- 1 scallion, both green and white parts, chopped
- 2 Tbsp. chopped fresh parsley
- 2 Tbsp. freshly squeezed lemon juice
- 1 Tbsp. chopped fresh thyme
- 1 tsp. chopped savory
- 1 tsp. chopped fresh oregano
- Water
- 1 cup fresh green beans, cut into 1-inch pieces
- Ground black pepper

Directions
1. Melt the butter in a pot.
2. Sauté the onion and garlic in the melted butter for 3 minutes or until the vegetables are softened.
3. Add the celery, cabbage, scallion, parsley, lemon juice, thyme, savory, and oregano to the pot; add enough water to cover the vegetables by 4 inches.
4. Bring the soup to a boil. Change the heat to low and simmer the soup for 25 minutes or until the vegetables are tender.
5. Add the green beans and simmer for 3 minutes.
6. Season with pepper.

Nutrition
- Calories: 33 -Fat: 1 g. -Carb: 6 g. -Phosphorus: 29 mg. -Potassium: 187 mg.
- Sodium: 20 mg. -Protein: 1 g.

39. Baked Haddock

Preparation time: 10 Minutes
Cooking time: 20 Minutes
Servings: 4

Ingredients

- ½ cup breadcrumbs
- 3 Tbsp. chopped fresh parsley
- 1 Tbsp lemon zest
- 1 tsp. chopped fresh thyme
- ¼ tsp. ground black pepper
- 1 Tbsp. melted unsalted butter
- 12 oz. Haddock fillets, deboned and skinned

Directions

1. Preheat the oven to 350°F.
2. In a bowl, stir together the parsley, breadcrumbs, lemon zest, thyme, and pepper until well combined.
3. Add the melted butter and toss until the mixture resembles coarse crumbs.
4. Place the haddock on a baking sheet and spoon the bread crumb mixture on top, pressing down firmly.
5. Bake the haddock in the oven for 20 minutes. You may wait until the fish is just cooked through and flakes off in chunks when pressed.

Nutrition

- Calories: 143
- Fat: 4 g.
- Carb: 10 g.
- Phosphorus: 216 mg.
- Potassium: 285 mg.
- Sodium: 281 mg.
- Protein: 16 g.

40. Herbed Chicken

Preparation time: 20 Minutes
Cooking time: 15 Minutes
Servings: 4

Ingredients
- 12 oz. boneless, skinless chicken breast, cut into eight strips
- 1 egg white
- 2 Tbsp. water, divided
- ½ cup breadcrumbs
- ¼ cup unsalted butter, divided
- Juice 1 lemon; Zest 1 lemon
- 1 Tbsp. fresh chopped basil
- 1 tsp. fresh chopped thyme
- Lemon slices, for garnish

Directions
1. Put the chicken strips between 2 sheets of plastic wrap and pound each flat with a rolling pin.
2. In a bowl, stick together the egg and 1 tbsp water.
3. Put the breadcrumbs in another bowl.
4. Cover the chicken strips, one at a time, in the egg then the breadcrumbs, and set the breaded strips aside on a plate.
5. In a large frypan over medium heat, thaw 2 tbsps. of the butter.
6. Cook the butter strips for 3 minutes, turning once, or until they are golden and cooked through. Transfer the chicken to a plate.
7. Add the lemon zest, lemon juice, basil, thyme and remaining 1 tbsp water to the skillet and stir until the mixture simmers.
8. Remove the sauce from the heat and mix in the remaining 2 tbsps. butter
9. Serve the chicken with the lemon sauce drizzled over the top and garnish with lemon slices.

Nutrition
- Calories: 255 -Fat: 14 g.
- Carb: 11 g. -Phosphorus: 180 mg. -Potassium: 321 mg. -Sodium: 261 mg. -Protein: 20 g.

41. Pesto Pork Chops

Preparation time: 20 Minutes
Cooking time: 20 Minutes
Servings: 4

Ingredients

- 4 (3-oz.) pork top-loin chops, boneless, fat trimmed
- 8 tsp. herb pesto
- ½ cup breadcrumbs
- 1 Tbsp. olive oil

Directions

1. Preheat the oven to 450°F.
2. Line a baking sheet with foil. Set aside.
3. Rub 1 tsp. of pesto evenly over both sides of each pork chop.
4. Lightly dredge each pork chop in the breadcrumbs.
5. Heat the oil in a skillet.
6. Brown the pork chops on each side for 5 minutes.
7. Place the pork chops on the baking sheet.
8. Bake for 10 minutes or until pork reaches 145°F in the center.

Nutrition

- Calories: 210
- Fat: 7 g.
- Carb: 10 g.
- Phosphorus: 179 mg.
- Potassium: 220 mg.
- Sodium: 148 mg.
- Protein: 24 g.

42. Vegetable Curry

Preparation time: 15 Minutes
Cooking time: 45 Minutes
Servings: 4
Ingredients

- 2 tsp. olive oil
- ½ sweet onion, diced
- 2 tsp. minced garlic
- 2 tsp. grated fresh ginger
- ½ eggplant, peeled and diced
- 1 carrot, peeled and diced
- 1 red bell pepper, diced
- 1 Tbsp. hot curry powder
- 1 tsp. ground cumin
- ½ tsp. coriander; Pinch cayenne pepper
- 1 ½ cups homemade vegetable stock
- 1 Tbsp. cornstarch; ¼ cup water

Directions

1. Heat the oil in a stockpot.
2. Sauté the ginger, garlic, and onion for 3 minutes or until they are softened.
3. Add the red pepper, carrots, and eggplant, and often stir for 6 minutes.
4. Stir in the cumin, curry powder, coriander, cayenne pepper, and vegetable stock.
5. Bring the curry to a boil and then lower the heat to low.
6. Simmer the curry for 30 minutes or until the vegetables are tender.
7. In a bowl, stir together the cornstarch and water.
8. Stir in the cornstarch mixture into the curry and simmer for 5 minutes or until the sauce has thickened.

Nutrition

- Calories: 100 -Fat: 3 g.
- Carb: 9 g. -Phosphorus: 28 mg. -Potassium: 180 mg. -Sodium: 218 mg. -Protein: 1 g.

43. Grilled Steak With Salsa

Preparation time: 20 Minutes
Cooking time: 15 Minutes
Servings: 4
Ingredients
For the salsa:

- 1 cup chopped English cucumber
- ¼ cup boiled and diced red bell pepper
- 1 scallion, both green and white parts, chopped
- 2 Tbsps. chopped fresh cilantro
- Juice 1 lime

For the steak:

- 4 (3-oz.) beef tenderloin steaks, room temperature
- Olive oil
- freshly ground black pepper

Directions

1. **To make the salsa:** In a bowl, combine the lime juice, cilantro, scallion, bell pepper, and cucumber. Set aside.
2. **To make the steak:** Preheat a barbecue to medium heat.
3. Rub the steaks all finished with oil and season with pepper.
4. Grill the steaks for around 5 minutes on each side for medium-rare or until the desired doneness.
5. Serve the steaks topped with salsa.

Nutrition

- Calories: 130
- Fat: 6 g. - Carb: 1 g.
- Phosphorus: 186 mg.
- Potassium: 272 mg.
- Sodium: 39 mg.
- Protein: 19 g.

44. Persian Chicken

Preparation time: 10 Minutes
Cooking time: 20 Minutes
Servings: 5

Ingredients
- ½ sweet onion, chopped
- ¼ cup lemon juice
- 1 Tbsp. dried oregano
- 1 tsp. minced garlic
- 1 tsp. sweet paprika
- ½ tsp. ground cumin
- ½ cup olive oil
- 5 boneless, skinless chicken thighs

Directions
1. Put the cumin, paprika, garlic, oregano, lemon juice, and onion in a food processor, and pulse to mix the ingredients.
2. Retain the motor running and add the olive oil until the mixture is even.
3. Put the chicken thighs in a large sealable freezer container and pour the sauce into the bag.
4. Seal the container and place it in the fridge, turning the bag 2 times for 2 hours.
5. Get rid of the thighs from the marinade and discard the extra marinade.
6. Preheat the barbecue to medium.
7. Grill the chicken for about 20 minutes, turning once, until it reaches 165°F.

Nutrition
- Calories: 321
- Fat: 21g
- Carb: 3 g.
- Phosphorus: 131 mg.
- Potassium: 220 mg.
- Sodium: 86 mg.
- Protein: 22 g.

45. Creamy Chicken With Cider

Preparation time: 5 Minutes
Cooking time: 25 Minutes
Servings: 8

Ingredients
- 4 bone-in chicken breasts
- 2 Tbsp. lightly salted butter
- ¾ cup apple cider vinegar
- ⅔ cup creamy unsweetened coconut milk or cream
- Kosher pepper

Directions
1. Thaw the butter in a skillet over medium heat.
2. Season the chicken with pepper and put it in the skillet. Cook over low heat for approx. 20 minutes.
3. Remove the chicken from the heat and set it aside in a dish.
4. In the same skillet, add the cider and bring to a boil until most of it has evaporated.
5. Add the coconut cream and let cook for 1 minute until slightly thickened.
6. Pour the cider cream over the cooked chicken and serve.

Nutrition
- Calories: 86.76
- Carbohydrate: 1.88 g.
- Protein: 1.5 g.
- Sodium: 93.52 mg.
- Potassium: 74.65 mg.
- Phosphorus: 36.54 mg.
- Dietary Fiber: 0.1 g.
- Fat: 8.21 g.

46. Exotic Palabok

Preparation time: 5 Minutes
Cooking time: 15 Minutes
Servings: 6
Ingredients

- 12 oz. rice noodles.
- 1 ½ cups medium shrimp, peeled and deveined
- ⅔ cup white onion, chopped
- 1 spring onion, sliced
- 1 garlic clove, minced
- 3 Tbsp. canola oil
- 1 lb. lean ground turkey
- 2 cups firm tofu, chopped
- 2 packs shrimp or ordinary gravy mix
- 5 hard-boiled eggs
- 1 lemon
- ½ cup pork rinds (optional)

Directions

1. Boil rice noodles until nice and soft. Keep aside.
2. Boil the peeled shrimp for 2–3 minutes in a pot with plain water.
3. In a wok or shallow pan, sauté the garlic and onion with the oil. Add ground turkey, tofu, and shrimp.
4. Dissolve the gravy mix in water or as per package instructions.
5. Combine the rice noodles, tofu, onions, and the gravy mix with ½ cup of pork rind (optional).
6. Slice the egg and lemons.
7. Serve with egg and lemons on top.

Nutrition

- Calories: 305 -Carbohydrate: 39.14 g.
- Protein: 17.6 g. -Sodium: 536 mg.
- Potassium: 243.52 mg. -Phosphorus: 180.41 mg. -Dietary Fiber: 0.9 g.

47. Vegetarian Gobi Curry

Preparation time: 5 Minutes
Cooking time: 15 Minutes
Servings: 8
Ingredients
- 2 cups cauliflower florets
- 2 Tbsp. unsalted butter
- 1 medium dry white onion, thinly chopped
- ½ cup green peas (frozen if wish)
- 1 tsp. fresh ginger, chopped
- ½ tsp. turmeric
- 1 tsp garam masala
- ¼ tsp. cayenne pepper
- 1 Tbsp. water

Directions
1. Warm a skillet over medium heat with the butter and sauté the onions until caramelized (golden brown).
2. Add the spices, e.g., ginger, garam masala turmeric, and cayenne.
3. Add the cauliflower and the (frozen) peas and stir.
4. Add the water and cover with a lid. Reduce the heat to a low temperature and let cook covered for 10 minutes.
5. Serve with white rice.

Nutrition
- Calories: 91.04 - Carbohydrate: 7.3 g.
- Protein: 2.19 g.
- Sodium: 39.38 mg.
- Potassium: 209.58 mg.
- Phosphorus: 42 mg.
- Dietary Fiber: 3 g.
- Fat: 6.4 g.

Chapter 11: Snacks

48. Peanut Butter Sandwich Snacks

Preparation time: 5 Minutes
Cooking time: 5 Minutes
Servings: 1
Ingredients
- 1 Tbsp peanut butter (powdered)
- 2¼ tsp water
- 6 crackers Crispbread, Whole Grain (34°), or similar product
- 1½ tsp chocolate syrup
- ¼ tsp Sprinkles, nonpareil

Directions
1. Mix the powdered peanut butter and water in a clean small bowl and stir until it becomes smooth.
2. Spread the peanut butter evenly over 3 crackers and top it with the remaining 3 crackers biscuit or bread.
3. Take half a tsp. of chocolate syrup and spread it over half the top of each cracker sandwich. Top chocolate syrup with sprinkles.

Nutrition
- Calories: 327
- Carbs: 30 g.
- Fat: 17.9 g.
- Protein: 15.0 g.

49. Peanut Butter Apple Slices

Preparation time: 10 Minutes
Cooking time: 10 Minutes
Servings: 4

Ingredients
- 2 pieces large apples
- ½ cup powdered peanut butter (reconstituted)
- 2 Tbsp. semi-sweet chocolate chips
- 2 Tbsp. slivered almonds
- 2 Tbsp. pecans (chopped)

Directions
1. Remove the core of the apple using a small paring knife or an apple corer
2. Slice the apples into thick rings.
3. Add the peanut butter over the apple slices.
4. Use chips and nuts for top-up

Nutrition
- Calories: 218
- Carbs: 31.3 g.
- Fat: 8.1 g.
- Protein: 11.6 g.

50. Baked Plantains

Preparation time: 5 Minutes
Cooking time: 35 Minutes
Servings: 2
Ingredients
- 2 medium-sized very overripe plantains
- Cooking spray olive oil
- Salt to taste

Directions
1. On a preheated oven at 350°F, line a baking sheet with a silicone mat or parchment paper and spray with olive oil or non-fat cooking spray.
2. Thinly slice plantains and place them on the baking sheet evenly, then lightly mist with olive oil or the non-fat cooking spray and sprinkle with a bit of salt.
3. For about 30–35 minutes, cook in the oven, flipping once about halfway through until they become golden and mostly crisp.

Nutrition
- Calories: 184
- Carbs: 47 g.
- Fat: 0.5 g.
- Protein: 2 g.

51. Strawberries and Cream Chocolate Cookie Sandwich

Preparation time: 5 Minutes
Cooking time: 5 Minutes
Servings: 1
Ingredients
- 2 Tbsp. topping (lite whipped)
- 1 medium strawberry (hulled, sliced)
- 2 square(s) Graham cracker(s) (chocolate variety)

Directions
1. Scoop whipped topping onto one square-shaped graham cracker.
2. Top it with sliced strawberries and place another cracker on top of that.

Nutrition
- Calories: 280
- Carbs: 37 g.
- Fat: 12 g.
- Protein: 5 g.

52. Mini Chocolate Chip Cookies

Preparation time: 10 Minutes
Cooking time: 6 Minutes
Servings: 48 Cookies

Ingredients
- 2 Tbsp butter (salted, softened)
- 2 tsp canola oil
- ½ cup(s) brown sugar (packed, dark-variety)
- 1 tsp vanilla extract
- ⅛ tsp table salt
- 1 large egg white(s)
- ¾ cup(s) all-purpose flour
- ¼ tsp. baking soda
- 3 oz., about ½ cup, chocolate chips (semi-sweet)

Directions
1. Prepare the oven by preheating it to 375°F.
2. Mix the butter, oil, and sugar in a medium bowl.
3. Add vanilla and egg white, then mix thoroughly to combine. Toss in some salt to taste.
4. Mix the flour and baking soda in a small bowl and stir them into the batter.
5. Add the chocolate chips to the batter and stir to distribute evenly throughout.
6. Put 48 ½ tsps. of dough onto 2 large nonstick baking sheets. Leave small spaces between the cookies.
7. Bake the cookies until they become golden around the edges, about 4–6 minutes.
8. Cool the baked cookies on a wire rack.

Nutrition
- Calories: 113.7
- Carbs: 16.4 g.
- Fat: 5.9 g.
- Protein: 0.6 g.

53. Chocolate-Peppermint Thins

Preparation time: 15 Minutes
Cooking time: 5 Minutes
Servings: 16
Ingredients
- 3 ½ oz. chocolate chunk (coarsely chopped)
- 16 item(s) chocolate wafer(s) (thin variety)
- 1 oz. candy cane (finely crushed)

Directions
1. Arrange a large baking sheet with parchment or paper wax and line cookies close together in a single layer.
2. At 5 seconds interval, melt chocolate in a microwavable bowl and stir between each interval until all but one or two pieces melted, then remove from microwave and stir until fully dissolved.
3. Put the melted chocolate in a plastic bag and cut off a corner; in a zig-zag pattern, pipe the chocolate over cookies and sprinkle with the crushed candy cane; keep it refrigerated until it's set for at least an hour or overnight. Serve as desired (1 cookie per serving)

Nutrition
- Calories: 175
- Carbs: 21 g.
- Fat: 5 g.
- Protein: 7 g.

54. Chocolate-Dipped Baby Bananas

Preparation time: 5 Minutes
Cooking time: 0 Minutes
Servings: 12
Ingredients

- 12 small baby-variety bananas (peeled)
- 3 oz. chocolate (semisweet, chopped)
- ¾ tsp. butter (unsalted)
- 2 tbsp. coconut (shredded, unsweetened)

Directions

1. Place a large baking sheet with wax paper and insert a wooden craft stick in one end of each banana.
2. Mix butter and chocolate in a medium microwave bowl, then microwave on high heat for about 1 minute.
3. Taking one banana after another, spoon the chocolate over the banana's cover and sprinkle it with coconut while it is on a baking sheet. Keep it refrigerated until the chocolate sets in about 15 minutes.
4. Serve as desired (1 banana per serving)

Nutrition

- Calories: 210
- Carbs: 31.2 g.
- Fat: 1 g.
- Protein: 5.4 g.

55. Fall Harvest Salad

Preparation time: 15 Minutes
Cooking time: 0 Minutes
Servings: 4

Ingredients

- 4–5 cups kale greens (baby variety)
- 1 piece large apple (thinly sliced)
- ⅓ cup sweet pumpkin seeds (toasted)

For dressing:

- 1 Tbsp olive oil
- 1 tbsp maple syrup
- 2 Tbsp red wine vinegar
- 1 piece shallot (minced)
- ¼ tsp cinnamon
- 1 tsp Dijon mustard
- Pepper and salt, to taste

Directions

1. Beat all the ingredients for the dressing together in a small bowl
2. Toss the ingredients for the salad in a large bowl
3. Pour the processed dressing over the salad and toss to coat evenly
4. This perfect dish is sure to impress your guests and compliment your holiday meal. Be careful not to lick the bowl.

Nutrition

- Calories: 175
- Carbs: 25.7 g.
- Fat: 7.6 g.
- Protein: 4.8 g.

56. Two-Ingredient Ice Cream Cupcake Bites

Preparation time: 5 Minutes
Cooking time: 12 Minutes
Servings: 12
Ingredients

- 6 bar(s) ice cream bars (WW Dark chocolate-raspberry)
- 10 Tbsp. white flour (self-rising)
- 4 Tbsp. whipped topping (light)
- ½ Tbsp. sprinkles (rainbow)

Directions

1. After preheating the oven to 350°F, coat 12 mini muffin holes with cooking spray
2. Drop the ice cream from the sticks into a large bowl and allow it to melt slightly, then add some white flour and stir until it is well-mixed.
3. Evenly fill prepared muffin holes with the mixture and bake until a tester inserted in the center of a cupcake comes out without anything sticking to it, about 10-12 minutes.
4. Allow the cupcakes to cool in the pan for a few minutes before taking them out. Collect the processed muffins from the pan and cool them completely.
5. Put 1 tsp. of whipped topping in each cooled cupcake and spread the sprinkles over the top.

Nutrition

- Calories: 109
- Carbs: 10 g.
- Fat: 8 g.
- Protein: 12 g.

57. Lemon Blueberry Cheesecake Yogurt Bark

Preparation time: 1 Hour and 15 Minutes
Cooking time: 0 Minutes
Servings: 12

Ingredients

- 1 cup Greek yogurt (plain non-fat)
- 1 Tbsp. agave nectar
- ½ tsp. lemon zest
- ½ tsp. lemon juice (fresh-squeezed)
- 1 cup blueberries (fresh)
- 3 squares (gluten-free if you like) Graham crackers (crushed into crumbs)

Directions

1. Line a 9x5-inch loaf pan with aluminum foil so that the foil hangs over the sides of the pan.
2. Mix the yogurt, lemon zest, agave nectar, and lemon juice in a small mixing bowl, then stir.
3. Turn in the blueberries gently with three Tbsp.s crushed graham cracker crumbs just until adequately mixed.
4. Evenly spread the mixture into the loaf pan you earlier prepared. Get the remaining cracker crumbs and sprinkle them over the top.
5. Use aluminum foil to cover the loaf pan and refrigerate for at least 1 hour; until it is frozen.
6. Once the mixture is frozen, remove the pan from the freezer and use overhanging foil as handles to lift the bark from the pan.
7. Put the frozen mixture on a cutting board and slice it into eight squares.
8. Cut each square diagonally, creating two triangles. (If the frozen dough is too difficult to cut, allow it to sit out at room temperature to soften. Alternatively, you can keep the knife inside hot water before cutting.)
9. Keep the cut portions in an airtight container inside the freezer until you are ready to serve. Allow the cut triangles to sit on the table at room temperature to soften slightly before serving if it is too frozen.

Nutrition

- Calories: 124 -Carbs: 12.7 g. -Fat: 0.2 g. -Protein: 18.2 g.

58. Dark Chocolate Avocado Mousse

Preparation time: 1 Hour and 10 Minutes
Cooking time: 0 Minutes
Servings: 2

Ingredients

- 1 large avocado (very ripe, peeled, and seeded)
- 2 oz. dark baking chocolate (70% cacao, melted)
- 2 Tbsp. cocoa powder (unsweetened)
- ¼ cup almond milk (unsweetened)
- 2 Tbsp. maple syrup
- ¼ tsp. pure vanilla extract
- A pinch cinnamon (ground)
- A pinch salt

Directions

1. Get a blender and put in avocado, maple syrup, melted chocolate, milk, cocoa powder, vanilla, cinnamon, and salt.
2. Process the content of the blender until you get a smooth and creamy mixture. To make the mousse thinner, add more milk or less milk for a thicker mousse.
3. Pour the mixture evenly into two small dessert glasses.
4. Chill it for at least 1 hour in the refrigerator before serving.

Nutrition

- Calories: 434
- Carbs: 53 g.
- Fat: 29 g.
- Protein: 6 g.

59. Hearty Chia and Blackberry Pudding

Preparation time: 45 Minutes
Cooking time: 0 Minutes
Servings: 2
Ingredients

- ¼ cup chia seeds
- ½ cup blackberries, fresh
- 1 tsp. liquid sweetener
- 1 cup coconut almond milk, full fat and unsweetened
- 1 tsp. vanilla extract

Directions

1. Take the vanilla, liquid sweetener, and coconut almond milk, and add to blender.
2. Process until thick.
3. Add in blackberries and chia and process until smooth.
4. Divide the mixture between cups and chill for 30 minutes.
5. Serve and enjoy!

Nutrition

- Calories: 437
- Fat: 38 g.
- Carbohydrates: 8 g.
- Protein: 8 g.

60. Special Cocoa Brownie Bombs

Preparation time: 15 Minutes
Cooking time: 25 Minutes
Servings: 12
Ingredients

- 2 Tbsp. grass-fed almond butter
- 1 whole egg
- 2 tsp. vanilla extract
- ¼ tsp. baking powder
- ⅓ cup heavy cream
- ¾ cup almond butter
- ¼ cocoa powder
- A pinch sunflower seeds

Directions

1. Break the eggs and whisk until smooth.
2. Add in all the wet ingredients and mix well.
3. Make the batter by mixing all the dry ingredients and sifting them into the wet ingredients.
4. Pour into a greased baking pan.
5. Bake for 25 minutes at 350°F or until a toothpick inserted in the middle comes out clean.
6. Let it cool, slice and serve.

Nutrition

- Total Carbs: 1 g.
- Fiber: 0 g.
- Protein: 1 g.
- Fat: 20 g.

61. Gentle Blackberry Crumble

Preparation time: 10 Minutes
Cooking time: 45 Minutes
Servings: 4
Ingredients
- ½ cup coconut flour
- ½ cup banana, peeled and mashed
- 6 Tbsp. water
- 3 cups fresh blackberries
- ½ cup arrowroot flour
- 1 ½ tsp. baking soda
- 4 Tbsp. almond butter, melted
- 1 Tbsp. fresh lemon juice

Directions

1. Preheat your oven to 300°F.
2. Take a baking dish and grease it lightly.
3. Take a bowl and mix all of the ingredients except the blackberries; mix well.
4. Place blackberries in the bottom of your baking dish and top with flour.
5. Bake for 40 minutes.
6. Serve and enjoy!

Nutrition
- Calories: 12
- Fat: 7 g.
- Carbohydrates: 10 g.
- Protein: 4 g.

62. Mini Minty Happiness

Preparation time: 2 Hours and 45 Minutes
Cooking time: 0 Minutes
Servings: 12

Ingredients

- 2 tsp. vanilla extract
- 1 ½ cups coconut oil
- 1 ¼ cups sunflower seed almond butter
- ½ cup dried parsley
- 1 tsp. peppermint extract
- A pinch sunflower seeds
- 1 cup dark chocolate chips Stevia, to taste

Directions

1. Melt together coconut oil and dark chocolate chips over a double boiler.
2. Take a food processor, add all the ingredients into it, and pulse until smooth.
3. Pour into round molds.
4. Let it freeze.

Nutrition

- Calories: 22
- Total Carbs: 7 g.
- Fiber: 1 g.
- Protein: 3 g.
- Fat: 25 g.

63. Astonishing Maple Pecan Bacon Slices

Preparation time: 10 Minutes
Cooking time: 25 Minutes
Servings: 12
Ingredients

- 2 Tbsp. sugar-free maple syrup
- 12 bacon slices
- Granulated Stevia, to taste
- 15–20 drops Stevia

For the coating:

- 4 Tbsp. dark cocoa powder
- ¼ cup pecans, chopped
- 15–20 drops Stevia

Directions

1. Take a baking tray and lay the bacon slices on it.
2. Rub with maple syrup and Stevia, flip the slices and do the same with the other side.
3. Bake for 10–15 minutes at 227°F.
4. After they've baked, drain the bacon grease.
5. To form a batter, mix the bacon grease, Stevia, and cocoa powder.
6. Dip the bacon slices into the batter and roll in the chopped pecans.
7. Allow to air dry until the chocolate hardens.

Nutrition

- Calories: 20
- Total Carbs: 1 g.
- Fiber: 0 g.
- Protein: 10 g.
- Fat: 11 g.

64. Generous Maple and Pecan Bites

Preparation time: 10 Minutes
Cooking time: 25 Minutes
Servings: 12
Ingredients

- 1 cup almond meal
- ½ cup coconut oil
- ½ cup flaxseed meal
- ½ cup sugar-free chocolate chips
- 2 cups pecans, chopped
- ½ cup sugar-free maple syrup
- 20–25 drops Stevia

Directions

1. Take a baking dish and spread the pecans.
2. Bake at 350°F until aromatic. This will usually take from 6–8 minutes.
3. Meanwhile, sift together all the dry ingredients.
4. Add the roasted pecans to the mix and mix them properly.
5. Add the coconut oil and maple syrup.
6. Stir to make a thick, sticky mixture.
7. Take a bread pan lined with parchment paper and pour the mixture into it.
8. Bake for about 18 minutes.
9. Slice and serve.

Nutrition

- Calories: 36
- Total Carbs: 6 g.
- Fiber: 0 g.
- Protein: 5 g.
- Fat: 30 g.

65. Carrot Ball Delight

Preparation time: 10 Minutes
Cooking time: 0 Minutes
Servings: 4

Ingredients
- 6 Medjool dates pitted
- 1 carrot, finely grated
- ¼ cup raw walnuts
- ¼ cup unsweetened coconut, shredded
- 1 tsp. nutmeg
- ⅛ tsp. sunflower seeds

Directions
1. Take a food processor and add dates, ¼ cup of grated carrots, sunflower seeds, coconut, and nutmeg.
2. Mix well and puree the mixture.
3. Add the walnuts and remaining ¼ cup of carrots.
4. Pulse the mixture until you have a chunky texture.
5. Form balls using your hand and roll them up in coconut.
6. Top with carrots and chill.
7. Enjoy!

Nutrition
- Calories: 326
- Fat: 16 g.
- Carbohydrates: 42 g.
- Protein: 3 g.

66. Awesome Brownie Muffins

Preparation time: 10 Minutes
Cooking time: 35 Minutes
Servings: 5
Ingredients
- 1 cup golden flaxseed meal
- ¼ cup cocoa powder
- 1 Tbsp. cinnamon
- ½ Tbsp. baking powder
- ½ tsp. sunflower seeds
- 1 whole large egg
- 2 Tbsp. coconut oil
- ¼ cup sugar-free caramel syrup
- ½ cup pumpkin puree
- 1 tsp. vanilla extract
- 1 tsp. apple cider vinegar
- ¼ cup almonds, slivered

Directions
1. Preheat your oven to 350°F.
2. Take a mixing bowl and add all of the listed ingredients and mix everything well.
3. Take your desired number of muffin tins and line them with paper liners.
4. Scoop the batter into the muffin tins, filling them with about ¼ of the liner.
5. Sprinkle a bit of almond on top.
6. Place them in your oven and bake for 15 minutes.
7. Serve warm.

Nutrition
- Calories: 55; Total Carbs: 16
- Fiber: 2 g.
- Protein: 3 g.
- Fat: 31 g.

67. Spice Friendly Muffins

Preparation time: 5 Minutes
Cooking time: 45 Minutes
Servings: 12

Ingredients
- ½ cup raw hemp hearts
- ½ cup flaxseeds
- ¼ cup chia seeds
- 2 Tbsp. Psyllium husk powder
- 1 Tbsp. cinnamon
- Stevia, to taste
- ½ tsp. baking powder
- ½ tsp. sunflower seeds
- 1 cup water

Directions
1. Preheat your oven to 350°F.
2. Line muffin tray with liners.
3. Take a large-sized mixing bowl and add all wet ingredients and mix well.
4. Keep stirring until the mixture has been thoroughly combined.
5. Take another bowl and add baking powder, spices and seeds.
6. Mix well.
7. Add the dry ingredients into the wet bowl and stir until well combined.
8. Divide the mixture amongst your muffin tins and bake for 45 minutes.
9. Enjoy!

Nutrition
- Calories: 36
- Total Carbs: 7 g.
- Fiber: 3 g.
- Protein: 6 g.
- Fat: 15 g.

68. Lime Grilled Pineapple

Preparation time: 10 Minutes
Cooking time: 10 Minutes
Servings: 8

Ingredients
- 1 Tbsp. lime juice
- 2 Tbsp. honey
- 1 Tbsp. olive oil
- 1 tsp. cinnamon, ground
- 1 pineapple, peeled and cut into medium pieces
- ¼ tsp. cloves, ground
- 1 Tbsp. dark rum
- 1 Tbsp. lime zest, grated

Directions
1. In a bowl, mix lime juice with honey, oil, cinnamon, and cloves, and whisk well.
2. Brush pineapple pieces with this marinade, skewer them and place on preheated grill over medium-high heat.
3. Cook for 5 minutes on each side, basting with the marinade from time to time.
4. Take them off heat, leave aside to cool down a bit, brush with rum, sprinkle lime zest, and serve warm or cold.

Nutrition
- Calories: 50
- Fat: 1 g.
- Fiber: 1 g.
- Carbs: 10 g.
- Protein: 0.5 g.

69. Sherry Hummus

Preparation time: 10 Minutes
Cooking time: 60 Minutes
Servings: 6

Ingredients
- ⅔ cup chickpeas, soaked overnight and drained
- 2 garlic cloves
- 3 cups water
- 1 bay leaf
- 1 Tbsp. olive oil
- A pinch salt
- 2 Tbsp. sherry vinegar
- ¾ cup green onions, chopped
- 1 tsp. cumin, ground
- 3 Tbsp. cilantro, chopped

Directions
1. Put the water in a pot, add a pinch of salt and chickpeas, and stir.
2. Add garlic and bay leaf as well, stir, bring to a simmer, cover partially, and cook for 1 hour.
3. Discard bay leaf and liquid but reserve ½ cup.
4. Transfer chickpeas to your food processor, add reserved liquid, green onions, vinegar, oil, garlic, cilantro, and cumin, and blend really well.
5. Transfer to a bowl and serve.

Nutrition
- Calories: 113
- Fat: 1 g.
- Fiber: 3 g.
- Carb: 10 g.
- Protein: 3 g.

70. Fruit Potpourri

Preparation time: 10 Minutes
Cooking time: 0 Minutes
Servings: 2
Ingredients
- 1 tsp. lime zest, grated
- 1 tsp. lime juice
- 6 oz. sugar-free and low-fat lemon yogurt
- 1 banana, peeled and cut in 4 medium wedges
- 4 strawberries
- 1 kiwi, peeled and cut into quarters
- 4 red grapes
- 4 pineapple pieces

Directions
1. Thread banana pieces, strawberries, grapes, pineapple chunks, and kiwi on skewers alternating them, and arrange on a platter.
2. In a bowl, mix lemon yogurt with lime zest and lime juice, whisk well, and keep in the fridge until you serve your fruit kebabs.

Nutrition
- Calories: 145
- Fat: 2 g.
- Fiber: 4 g.
- Carbs: 34 g.
- Protein: 4 g.

71. Citrus Fruit Salsa

Preparation time: 2 Hours and 10 Minutes
Cooking time: 12 Minutes
Servings: 10

Ingredients
- 1 Tbsp. brown sugar
- 8 whole-wheat tortillas, cut into medium pieces
- ½ Tbsp. cinnamon powder
- 3 cups mixed apples with oranges and grapes
- 1 Tbsp. agave nectar
- 2 Tbsp. sugar-free jam
- 2 Tbsp. orange juice

Directions
1. In a bowl, combine mixed fruits with agave nectar, jam, and orange juice, toss well, cover, and keep in the fridge for 2 hours.
2. Meanwhile, spread tortilla pieces on a lined baking sheet, sprinkle cinnamon powder and sugar all over them and bake in the oven at 350°F for 12 minutes.
3. Divide fruits salsa into bowls and serve with tortilla chips on the side.

Nutrition
- Calories: 110
- Fat: 2 g.
- Fiber: 2 g.
- Carbs: 20 g.
- Protein: 2 g.

Chapter 12: Dinner

72. Apple Glazed Chicken With Spinach

Preparation time: 5 Minutes
Cooking time: 5 Minutes
Servings: 2
Ingredients
- ¼ cup apple jelly
- 1 Tbsp. reduced-sodium soy sauce
- 2 tsp. snipped fresh thyme
- ½ tsp. finely shredded lemon peel
- ½ tsp. grated fresh ginger
- 2 (4 oz.) skinless, boneless chicken breast halves
- ⅛ tsp. salt
- ⅛ tsp. black pepper
- Nonstick cooking spray
- 1 medium apple, cored and coarsely chopped
- ¼ cup sliced onion
- 1 clove garlic, minced
- 6 cups packaged prewashed fresh spinach

Directions
1. To make the glaze, mix together ginger, lemon peel, thyme, soy sauce, and apple jelly in a small microwave-safe bowl. Microwave for 60–90 seconds on 100% power (high) without cover or just until the jelly melts, mixing once. Set aside 2 tbsp. of the glaze.
2. Season with pepper and salt the chicken. On the unheated rack of a broiler pan, put the chicken, then broil for 12–15 minutes, placed 4–5 inches from the heat source or until the chicken has no visible pink color and becomes tender, flipping once halfway through the broiling process, then brush it with the leftover glaze during the final 5 minutes of broiling. Get rid of the leftover glaze that was used as a brush-on.
3. In the meantime, use nonstick cooking spray to coat an unheated big nonstick saucepan, then preheat it on medium heat. Add garlic, onion and apple into the hot saucepan, then let it cook

and stir for 3 minutes. Mix in the reserved 2 tbsp. of glaze, then boil. Add spinach, then toss just until it wilts.
4. To serve, halve the chicken breast crosswise into 6–8 pieces. Distribute the spinach mixture among the 2 dinner plates, then put the sliced chicken on top.

Nutrition
- Calories: 312
- Total Fat: 2 g.
- Saturated Fat: 0 g.
- Fiber: 5 g.
- Total Carbohydrate: 46 g.
- Protein: 30 g.
- Sodium: 555 mg.
- Cholesterol: 66 mg.
- Sugar: 31 g.

73. BBQ Ranch Wraps

Preparation time: 5 Minute
Cooking time: 0 Minutes
Servings: 4

Ingredients

- 2 Tbsp. bottled reduced-fat ranch salad dressing
- 1 Tbsp. light mayonnaise dressing or salad dressing
- 2 cups packaged shredded broccoli (broccoli slaw mix)
- 4 (8-inch) whole-grain flour tortillas
- 2 Tbsp. bottled barbecue sauce
- 8 oz. cooked chicken breast or turkey breast, shredded

Direction

1. Mix dressings together until smooth.
2. Cover the broccoli with the dressing mix and the chicken with barbecue sauce.
3. Scoop chicken and broccoli in the tortillas and serve.

Nutrition

- Calories: 279
- Total Fat: 7 g.
- Saturated Fat: 1 g.
- Cholesterol: 51 g.
- Total Carbohydrate: 31 g.
- Sugar: 5 g.
- Protein: 23 g.
- Sodium: 589 mg.
- Fiber: 3 g.

74. BLT Cups

Preparation time: 15 Minutes
Cooking time: 5 Minutes
Servings: 12

Ingredients

- 1 Tbsp. olive oil, or as needed
- 40 (16 oz.) packages wonton wrappers
- 8 strips cooked bacon, crumbled
- 4 plum tomatoes, chopped
- 1 cup shredded lettuce
- ½ cup light mayonnaise
- 1 Tbsp. honey mustard
- 3 green onions, chopped

Directions

1. Set an oven to preheat at 190°C (375°F). Use olive oil to grease the 40 mini muffin cups.
2. In each of the prepared muffin cups, press one wonton wrapper, pressing against the sides and bottom of the cup.
3. Bake in the oven for about 4 minutes until crisp and corners turn brown. Let it cool.
4. In a bowl, mix together the honey mustard, mayonnaise, lettuce, tomatoes and bacon until blended well. Fill every wonton with bacon mixture and put green onion on each top.

Nutrition

- Calories: 4476
- Total Fat: 33.1 g.
- Sodium: 8972 mg.
- Total Carbohydrate: 867.5 g.
- Cholesterol: 154 mg.
- Protein: 152.2 g.

75. Baked Beans With Ground Beef

Preparation time: 25 Minutes
Cooking time: 15 Minutes
Servings: 6

Ingredients

- 1 Tbsp. extra-virgin olive oil
- 1 medium onion, chopped
- 1 lb. lean ground beef
- 2 (15 oz) cans no-salt-added navy beans, rinsed
- 1 cup water
- ¾ cup ketchup
- ¼ cup molasses
- 1 tsp. Dijon mustard
- ½ tsp. garlic powder
- ¼ tsp. salt
- ¼ cup chopped fresh chives for garnish

Directions

1. In a big saucepan, heat the oil on medium-high heat, then add the ground beef and onion.
2. Let it cook for about 5 minutes, mix and crumble the beef using a wooden spoon until the beef has no visible pink color anymore and the onion becomes tender.
3. Add the salt, garlic powder, mustard, molasses, ketchup, water, and beans, then simmer. Lower the heat to medium and let it cook and stir for 5–8 minutes until the mixture becomes slightly thick and bubbly.
4. Put chives on top to garnish, if preferred.

Nutrition

- Calories: 346 -Total Carbohydrate: 41 g.-Protein: 23 g.-Total Fat: 10 g.
- Saturated Fat: 3 g.
- Sodium: 525 mg.
- Fiber: 7 g.-Cholesterol: 49 mg.
- Sugar: 18 g.

76. Baked Chicken Taquitos

Preparation time: 10 Minutes
Cooking time: 15 Minutes
Servings: 2

Ingredients

- 1 cup shredded cooked chicken breast
- ¼ cup shredded reduced-fat cheddar cheese (1 oz.)
- 2 Tbsp. taco sauce
- ½ tsp. ground cumin
- 4 6-inch corn tortillas

Directions

1. Set an oven to preheat to 425°F. Line parchment paper on a baking tray, then put it aside.
2. To make the filling mix together the cumin, taco sauce, cheese, and chicken in a medium bowl, then put aside.
3. Pile the wrap and tortillas in damp paper towels. Let it microwave for 40 seconds on 100% power (high) or until it becomes soft and warm. Spread ¼ of the filling onto the bottom third of each tortilla, then roll up the tortilla tightly. Put it on the prepped baking tray, seam sides down.
4. Let it bake for 15 minutes or until the edges of the tortillas begin to brown.

Nutrition

- Calories: 242
- Cholesterol: 70 mg.
- Protein: 27 g.
- Total Carbohydrate: 17 g.
- Sugar: 3 g.
- Total Fat: 7 g.
- Saturated Fat: 3 g.
- Sodium: 239 mg.
- Fiber: 3 g.

77. Baked Fish Tacos With Avocado

Preparation time: 20 Minutes
Cooking time: 15 Minutes
Servings: 4
Ingredients

- 1 Tbsp. avocado oil
- 2 tsp. no-salt-added Mexican-style seasoning blend
- ½ tsp. salt
- 1 lb. flaky white fish fillets, such as cod, haddock, or mahi-mahi, cut into 8 or 16 pieces
- 1 avocado, cut into 16 slices
- ½ cup Pico de Gallo
- 8 corn tortillas, warmed

Directions

1. Set an oven to preheat to 400°F. Use cooking spray to coat a big rimmed baking tray.
2. In a medium bowl, stir together the salt, seasoning blend and oil, then add the fish and toss until coated. Move to the prepped baking tray and let it bake for around 10 minutes (It depends on the thickness) until the fish flakes easily.
3. Put 1 tbsp. of Pico de Gallo, 2 avocado slices and 1–2 pieces of fish in each tortilla to assemble the tacos.

Nutrition

- Calories: 296
- Saturated Fat: 2 g.
- Cholesterol: 45 g.
- Sugar: 3 g.
- Protein: 19 g.
- Total Fat: 13 g.
- Total Carbohydrate: 29 g.
- Sodium: 521 mg.
- Fiber: 6 g.

78. Beef and Vegetables in Peanut Sauce

Preparation time: 10 Minutes - **Cooking time:** 10 Minutes
Servings: 2

Ingredients

- ½ cup cold water
- 3 Tbsp. powdered peanut butter, such as PB2 brand
- 1 Tbsp. reduced-sodium teriyaki sauce
- 1 Tbsp. cider vinegar
- 2 tsp. honey
- ¼ tsp. ground ginger
- ¼ tsp. crushed red pepper
- Nonstick cooking spray
- 6 oz. boneless beef sirloin, cut into thin bite-size strips
- 1 clove garlic, minced
- 1 cup fresh snow pea pods, trimmed
- ½ cup purchased shredded carrots
- ½ 8.8-oz. pouch cooked brown rice (1 cup), heated according to package directions

Directions

1. To make the peanut sauce, stir peanut butter powder and cold water together in a small saucepan until the powder is dissolved. Stir in crushed red pepper, ginger, honey, vinegar, and teriyaki sauce, then boil, occasionally stirring. Gently simmer without a cover for 1–2 minutes until sauce thickens, then put aside.
2. Use cooking spray to coat a big nonstick skillet and heat over medium-high heat, then add the garlic and beef, cook while stirring for 2 minutes. Add carrots and pea pods, and cook, stirring for 2 more minutes until vegetables become tender-crisp.
3. Add peanut sauce and stir to coat, then heat through if needed.
4. Serve vegetable and beef mixture over hot brown rice.

Nutrition

- Calories: 353 -Fiber: 3 g.-Cholesterol: 34 mg.-Total Carbohydrate: 36 g.
- Sugar: 10 g.-Total Fat: 12 g.-Saturated Fat: 4 g.-Sodium: 345 mg.-Protein: 26 g.

79. Black Bean Queso Wraps

Preparation time: 20 Minutes
Cooking time: 10 Minutes
Servings: 4

Ingredients

- ½ cup chopped red sweet pepper
- ¼ cup chopped poblano chile pepper (see Tip)
- 2 tsp. canola oil
- ⅓ cup thinly sliced green onions
- ⅓ cup canned reduced-sodium black beans, rinsed and drained
- ⅓ cup frozen whole-kernel corn, thawed
- 2 Tbsp. snipped fresh cilantro
- 2 Tbsp. salsa Verde
- 4 8-inch whole-wheat low-carb flour tortillas
- 1 cup shredded queso Oaxaca or Monterey Jack cheese (4 oz.)
- Nonstick cooking spray

Directions

1. Cook the poblano pepper and sweet pepper in a medium skillet with hot oil over moderate heat for 3–5 minutes, stirring occasionally or until the ingredients are crisp-tender. Mix in green onions. Remove the mixture from heat and stir in cilantro, corn, salsa Verde, and beans.
2. Put the tortillas between the paper towels. Place it inside the microwave and heat on 100 percent power (high) for 20–40 seconds or until warm. Scoop the bean mixture into the tortillas, placing it below its centers. Top the mixture with cheese. Fold the bottom edge of each tortilla up and over the filling. Also, fold the opposite sides and roll it up starting from the bottom. Use a cooking spray to lightly coat the outer part of the wraps.
3. Set the Panini press to preheat. Arrange the wraps in the press, half at a time if needed. Cover and allow them to cook for 2–3 minutes or until the fillings are heated through and the tortillas are toasted. You can also use a preheated grill pan or skillet to cook the tortillas. Place the pan over medium heat and arrange the wraps in the pan, half at a time if needed. Weight down with a heavy skillet and let them cook for 2–3 minutes or until the wrap is toasted. Flip

the wraps and weight down again. Let them cook for 2–3 more minutes or until the fillings are heated through and the wrap is toasted.

Nutrition
- Calories: 233
- Total Fat: 12 g.
- Fiber: 14 g.
- Cholesterol: 24 mg.
- Total Carbohydrate: 28 g.
- Protein: 17 g.
- Saturated Fat: 0 g.
- Sodium: 388 mg.
- Sugar: 3 g.

80. Broccoli and Cauliflower Sauté

Preparation time: 4 Minutes
Cooking time: 8 Minutes
Servings: 4
Ingredients

- 2 tsp. olive oil
- 1 cup broccoli florets
- 1 cup cauliflower florets
- 1 clove garlic, thinly sliced
- ¼ cup dry white wine or reduced-sodium chicken broth
- 3 Tbsp. water
- ⅛ tsp. salt
- ⅛ tsp. ground black pepper

Directions

1. Heat oil over medium-high heat in a big skillet. Put in garlic, cauliflower, and broccoli, then cook for 2 minutes, mixing occasionally. Put in pepper, salt, water, and wine carefully; decrease the heat to low. Cover and cook for 2 minutes.
2. Uncover; turn heat up to medium. Cook until vegetables are tender, about 2 minutes.

Nutrition

- Calories: 47
- Saturated Fat: 0 g.
- Fiber: 1 g.
- Cholesterol: 0 g.
- Total Carbohydrate: 4 g.
- Sugar: 1 g.
- Protein: 1 g.
- Total Fat: 2 g.
- Sodium: 88 mg.

81. Buffalo Deviled Eggs

Preparation time: 25 Minutes
Cooking time: 5 Minutes
Servings: 8
Ingredients

- 8 hard-boiled eggs, halved lengthwise with yolks and whites separated
- ¼ cup Greek yogurt
- 1 stalk celery, minced
- 2 Tbsp. minced Anaheim chile pepper
- 2 Tbsp. mayonnaise
- 1 ½ Tbsp. Dijon mustard
- 1 Tbsp. hot Buffalo wing sauce (such as Frank's® REDHOT Buffalo Wing Sauce), or to taste
- ¼ tsp. garlic salt
- ¼ tsp. onion powder
- ¼ tsp. ground black pepper
- ¼ tsp. paprika
- 2 Tbsp. finely grated Cheddar cheese, or more to taste

Directions

1. In a bowl, whisk together paprika, black pepper, onion powder, garlic salt, Buffalo wing sauce, mustard, mayonnaise, Anaheim pepper, yogurt, celery, and egg yolks with a fork until the mixture is smooth and creamy. Toss in Cheddar cheese.
2. On a dish, put the egg white halves. Use the egg yolk mixture to put evenly into each egg white half.

Nutrition

- Calories: 126
- Total Fat: 9.5 g.
- Sodium: 282 mg.
- Total Carbohydrate: 2.4 g.
- Cholesterol: 217 mg.
- Protein: 7.4 g.

82. Cajun Shrimp Grill Packets With Tomatoes Okra

Preparation time: 15 Minutes
Cooking time: 12 Minutes
Servings: 6

Ingredients

- 1 lb. raw large shrimp (26-30 per pound), peeled and deveined
- 5 cups whole okra, trimmed
- 5 cups cherry tomatoes
- 1 large yellow onion, sliced
- 3 Tbsp. extra-virgin olive oil
- 2 cloves garlic, minced
- 2 tsp. Cajun seasoning

Directions

1. Preheat the grill over medium-high. Cut six 14-inch lengths of heavy-duty foil. Use cooking spray to coat 1 side of each piece of foil.
2. In a large bowl, mix Cajun seasoning shrimp, garlic, okra, onion, oil, and tomatoes. Mix to coat well. Separate the mixture evenly into the foil sheets (put on the side that is covered with cooking spray) and layout the shrimp over the other ingredients. Bring together the long ends of every foil piece, and then fold up its open sides to shape into a packet.
3. Transfer the packets onto the grill. Cook for about 12 minutes until the shrimp is opaque and the veggies become tender.

Nutrition

- Calories: 175
- Total Fat: 8 g.
- Saturated Fat: 1 g.
- Fiber: 4 g.
- Sugar: 5 g.
- Sodium: 484 mg.
- Cholesterol: 95 mg.
- Total Carbohydrate: 14 g.
- Protein: 13 g.

83. Chicken Spring Vegetable Tortellini Salad

Preparation time: 30 Minutes
Cooking time: 15 Minutes
Servings: 6

Ingredients

- 1 lb. boneless, skinless chicken breast
- 2 bay leaves
- 6 cups water
- 1 (20 oz.) package fresh cheese tortellini
- ½ cup peas, fresh or frozen
- ¼ cup creamy salad dressing such as ranch or peppercorn
- 2 Tbsp. red-wine vinegar
- 5 Tbsp. chopped fresh herbs, such as basil, dill, and/or chives, divided
- ½ cup chopped marinated artichokes plus 2 Tbsp.s marinade, divided
- ½ cup julienned radishes
- 1 cup pea shoots or baby arugula
- 2 Tbsp. sunflower seeds

Directions

1. Mix bay leaves, water and chicken in a large saucepan, and bring the mixture to a boil over high heat. Adjust the heat to low and cover the pan. Allow the chicken to simmer for 10–12 minutes until an inserted instant-read thermometer in the thickest part of the chicken reads 165°F. Place the cooked chicken into the clean cutting board and allow it to cool.
2. Discard the bay leaves. Add tortellini into the pot and bring it back to a boil. Cook for about 3 minutes, occasionally stirring until the tortellini are just tender. Stir in peas and cook for 60 seconds more. Drain and wash with cold water.
3. In a large bowl, mix vinegar, artichoke marinade, dressing and 3 tbsp. of herbs. Shred the chicken and add them to the dressing. Stir in peas, radishes, tortellini and pea shoots (or arugula) until combined. Sprinkle sunflower seeds and the remaining 2 tbsp. of herbs on top of the salad before serving.

Nutrition

- Calories: 357
- Cholesterol: 47 mg.-Sugar: 3 g.-Saturated Fat: 3 g.
- Sodium: 452 g.-Protein: 24 g.-Total Fat: 13 g.-Fiber: 4 g.-Total Carbohydrate: 36 g.

84. Chicken Honey Nut Stir Fry

Preparation time: 5 Minutes
Cooking time: 5 Minutes
Servings: 1

Ingredients

- 2 tsp. vegetable oil
- ¼ cup carrot, sliced diagonally
- ¼ cup chopped celery
- 8 oz. skinless, boneless chicken breast halves, cut into 1-inch pieces
- ¼ cup orange juice
- 1 tsp. cornstarch
- 1 Tbsp. reduced-sodium soy sauce
- 1 tsp. honey
- ¼ tsp. grated fresh ginger
- 2 Tbsp. cashews
- 2 Tbsp. thinly sliced green onion
- ⅔ cup hot cooked brown rice

Directions

1. Heat 1 tsp. oil over high heat using a big skillet or a wok, and add the celery and carrot, then stir-fry the vegetables for 2 minutes. Add remaining 1 tsp. oil and the chicken, then stir-fry until the chicken is done, about 3–5 minutes.
2. In a small bowl, whisk cornstarch and orange juice together, then add ginger, honey and soy sauce, whisking to mix well. Add to the chicken mixture in the wok and cook while stirring over medium heat until it thickens; cook for 1 more minute. Top with green onion and cashews, then serve over hot brown rice.

Nutrition

- Calories: 336 -Cholesterol: 73 mg.-Sugar: 8 g.-Protein: 28 g.-Total Fat: 12 g.-Fiber: 2 g.
- Saturated Fat: 2 g.
- Sodium: 353 mg.
- Total Carbohydrate: 28g.

85. Curried Chicken With Cabbage, Apple and Onion

Preparation time: 15 Minutes
Cooking time: 15 Minutes
Servings: 4

Ingredients

- 1 tsp. curry powder
- ¼ tsp. salt
- ¼ tsp. ground black pepper
- 4 skinless, boneless chicken breast halves (1 to 1 ¼ lb. total)
- 2 tsp. olive oil
- 2 tsp. butter
- 1 medium onion, sliced and separated into rings
- 3 cups shredded cabbage
- 2 red-skin cooking apples (such as Rome or Jonathan), cored and thinly sliced
- ½ cup apple juice

Directions

1. Mix pepper, salt and ½ tsp. of the curry powder in a small bowl. Drizzle the spice mixture evenly atop the chicken. Rub with your fingers.
2. Over medium-high heat, heat oil in a large nonstick skillet, and then add chicken. Cook for about 8–12 minutes, flipping once, or until no pink color remains (170°F). Place the chicken onto a platter. Cover to keep the chicken warm.
3. Melt butter in the hot skillet and add onion. Cook for about 5 minutes while stirring often or until the onions become tender. Mix in apple juice, apple and cabbage. Drizzle the remaining ½ tsp. curry powder on top. Cook for about 3–4 minutes while stirring often or until the vegetables and apples become tender.
4. To serve, separate cabbage and chicken mixture into four dinner plates.

Nutrition

- Calories: 237 -Total Fat: 6 g.-Saturated Fat: 2 g.-Sugar: 13 g.-Cholesterol: 71 mg.
- Total Carbohydrate: 19 g.-Protein: 27 g.-Sodium: 231 mg.-Fiber: 4 g.

86. Curried Turkey Cutlets With Dried Apricots

Preparation time: 15 Minutes - **Cooking time:** 5 Minutes
Servings: 4 - **Ingredients**

- 2 tsp. extra-virgin olive oil; ½ cup finely chopped onion
- 3 cloves garlic, minced
- 1 Tbsp. minced fresh ginger
- ¼ tsp. salt, or to taste
- ¾ cup apple or pineapple juice
- ½ cup dried apricots, chopped
- 1 tsp. cornstarch mixed with 1 Tbsp. cold water
- 4 scallions, thinly sliced
- 1 lb. turkey cutlets, cut into four portions (see Ingredient note)
- ¼ cup low-fat plain yogurt
- Freshly ground pepper, to taste
- 2 Tbsp. slivered fresh mint (optional)
- 1–2 teaspoons curry powder

Directions

1. Pat the turkey cutlets dry with the paper towels; season with pepper and salt. Heat the oil in a big nonstick skillet on medium-high heat. Put in the turkey and cook 2–3 minutes on each side till not pink in the middle anymore and brown on both sides. Move into the dish and set aside.
2. Place the onion into pan; cook, mixing for 60 seconds. Put in the curry, ginger and garlic; cook, whisking roughly half a minute or till becoming fragrant. Place in the apricots and juice; simmer. Cook for around 3 minutes or till liquid decreases a bit and apricots are plump.
3. Put the cornstarch mixture into the pan and cook, mixing continuously, roughly 60 seconds or till becoming thick. Bring any accumulated juices and turkey back to the pan. Cook, flipping cutlets several times, 1–2 minutes or till becoming thoroughly heated and coated. Mix in the scallions and mint (if using). Serve instantly with a dollop of the yogurt.

Nutrition

- Calories: 239 -Protein: 30 g.-Total Carbohydrate: 23 g.-Sugar: 15 g.-Saturated Fat: 1 g.
- Sodium: 275 mg.-Fiber: 3 g.-Cholesterol: 46 mg.-Total Fat: 3 g.

87. Easy Butternut Squash Soup

Preparation time: 20 Minutes - **Cooking time:** 5 Minutes
Servings: 4 - **Ingredients**

- 1 (12 oz.) package refrigerated cubed butternut squash, such as Green Giant brand or Marketside (Walmart brand)
- ½ cup finely chopped onion
- 2 Tbsp. unsalted butter
- 1 (14.5 oz.) can reduced-sodium chicken broth
- 1 (12 fluid oz.) can fat-free evaporated milk
- 1 tsp. packed brown sugar
- ½ tsp. kosher salt
- ½ tsp. ground nutmeg
- ¼ tsp. ground white pepper (more if desired)
- Fresh thyme sprigs (optional)
- Freshly grated nutmeg (optional)

Directions

1. Put butternut squash package contents and 2 tbsp. water in a 2-qt. microwave-safe baking dish that has a lid; cover, microwave for 3 minutes on high/100% powder. Mix; microwave for 3 minutes more on high/100% power again. Mix again. Microwave for 2 minutes more till squash is very tender on high/100% powder. Mash the squash with a potato masher/pastry blender.
2. Meanwhile, cook onion in the hot butter till tender in a medium heavy saucepan, frequently mixing.
3. Process/blend white pepper, ½ tsp. ground nutmeg, salt, brown sugar, evaporated milk, broth, mashed squash and cooked onions, covered, till smooth in a food processor/blender. Put the soup back into the saucepan; mix and cook on medium-high heat to heat through. Garnish with freshly grated nutmeg and thyme if desired.

Nutrition

- Calories: 185 -Total Fat: 6 g.-Sodium: 560 mg.-Fiber: 2 g.-Cholesterol: 15 mg.
- Saturated Fat: 4 g.-Total Carbohydrate: 25 g.-Sugar: 15 g.-Protein: 8 g.

88. Easy Deviled Eggs

Preparation time: 20 Minutes
Cooking time: 10 Minutes
Servings: 24

Ingredients

- 12 large eggs
- ¼ cup nonfat plain Greek yogurt
- ¼ cup mayonnaise
- 1 Tbsp. minced shallot
- 2 tsp. Dijon mustard
- 1 tsp. white-wine vinegar
- ¼ tsp. salt
- ¼ tsp. ground pepper

Directions

1. In a saucepan, put eggs and fill them with water. Simmer it over medium-high heat. Lower the heat to low and simmer at its barest for 10 minutes. Take away from heat, discard the hot water, and use ice-cold water to cover the eggs. Let sit until cool enough to handle.
2. Remove the shell and use a sharp knife slice into two lengthwise. Carefully scoop out the yolks and put them in a food processor. Add pepper, salt, vinegar, mustard, shallot, mayonnaise, and yogurt, and blend until smooth.
3. Stuff the egg white halves with 1 tbsp. of the filling.

Nutrition

- Calories: 47
- Total Fat: 3 g.-Fiber: 0 g.
- Cholesterol: 94 mg.
- Protein: 3 g.
- Saturated Fat: 1 g.
- Sodium: 78 mg.
- Total Carbohydrate: 1 g.
- Sugar: 1 g.

89. Easy Grilled Zucchini

Preparation time: 10 Minutes
Cooking time: 10 Minutes
Servings: 4

Ingredients
- 1 Tbsp. olive oil
- 3 zucchinis, sliced ¼-inch thick, lengthwise
- 1 Tbsp. grill seasoning

Directions
1. Preheat the grill for medium heat, then lightly grease the grate with oil.
2. Sprinkle zucchini slices with olive oil on both sides and add grill seasoning to taste.
3. Grill zucchinis on preheated grill for 3–4 minutes on each side or until tender.

Nutrition
- Calories: 58
- Cholesterol: 0 mg.
- Protein: 1.9 g.
- Total Fat: 3.7 g.
- Sodium: 381 mg.
- Total Carbohydrate: 5.7 g.

90. Farfalle With Tuna, Lemon, and Fennel

Preparation time: 5 Minutes - **Cooking time:** 10 Minutes
Servings: 4 - **Ingredients**

- 6 oz. dried whole-grain farfalle (bow-tie) pasta
- 1 (5 oz.) can solid white tuna (packed in oil)
- Olive oil (optional)
- 1 cup fennel, thinly sliced (1 medium bulb)
- 2 cloves garlic, minced
- ½ tsp. crushed red pepper
- ¼ tsp salt
- 2 (14.5 oz.) cans no-salt-added diced tomatoes, undrained
- 2 Tbsp. snipped fresh Italian (flat-leaf) parsley
- 1 tsp. lemon peel, finely shredded

Directions

1. Follow the package directions to cook the pasta. Make sure to omit the salt. Drain. Place the pasta back into the pan and cover it to keep warm. In the meantime, drain the tuna and reserve oil. Add more oil to have a total of 3 tbsp. if necessary. Flake the tuna and then put it aside.
2. Heat 3 tbsp. of the reserved oil in a medium saucepan over medium heat. Add the fennel and cook it for 3 minutes while occasionally stirring. Add the salt, crushed red pepper and garlic. Cook and stir the mixture for about 1 minute or until the garlic is golden.
3. Mix in tomatoes. Bring the mixture to a boil. Lower the heat and simmer without a cover for 5–6 minutes or until the mixture begins to thicken. Mix in tuna and simmer without the lid for 1 more minute or until the tuna is heated through.
4. Pour tuna mixture all over the pasta. Mix it gently until well combined. Sprinkle lemon peel and parsley over each of the servings.

Nutrition

- Calories: 356 - Sodium: 380 mg.-Cholesterol: 11 mg.-Total Fat: 14 g.
- Saturated Fat: 2 g.-Fiber: 9 g.-Total Carbohydrate: 43 g.-Sugar: 8 g.-Protein: 17 g.

91. Fresh Sweet Corn Salad

Preparation time: 10 Minutes
Cooking time: 5 Minutes
Servings: 4

Ingredients

- 4 medium ears fresh corn, husked, or 10 oz. frozen whole-kernel corn, thawed
- 1 tsp. olive oil
- 1 cup thin strips orange bell pepper
- 1 cup thinly sliced red onion
- ½ tsp. kosher salt
- ¼ tsp. ground pepper
- 2 Tbsp. thinly sliced fresh basil for garnish

Directions

1. Chop off corn kernels from the cobs to have two cups.
2. Over medium heat, heat oil in a 10-inch skillet, then add the onion, corn and bell pepper. Cook while stirring for about 5 minutes until the onion and bell pepper become tender-crisp. Season with pepper and salt.
3. You can serve the salad chilled or warm. (Drain the vegetables before you chill.) If desired, sprinkle with basil before serving.

Nutrition

- Calories: 104
- Cholesterol: 0 mg.
- Protein: 3 g.
- Sodium: 155 mg.
- Fiber: 3 g.
- Sugar: 8 g.
- Total Carbohydrate: 21 g.

92. Fresh Tomato Soup

Preparation time: 20 Minutes
Cooking time: 6 Minutes
Servings: 6
Ingredients
- 2 lb. tomatoes, cored and seeded (see Tip)
- 1 ½ cups coarsely chopped red sweet peppers
- 1 cup reduced-sodium vegetable or chicken broth
- ¼ cup chopped sweet onion
- ¼ cup snipped fresh basil
- 2 Tbsp. heavy cream
- 1 Tbsp. honey
- Grilled Cheese Croutons (optional)

Directions
1. In batches, combine tomatoes, onion, broth, basil and peppers in a food processor or blender until smooth. In a large pot, put the mixture.
2. Over medium heat, cook for 5–6 minutes or until it is heated through. Mix in honey and cream. If preferred, top servings with basil leaves and Grilled Cheese Crouton. Enjoy warm.

Nutrition
- Calories: 69
- Total Carbohydrate: 11 g.
- Saturated Fat: 1 g.
- Fiber: 2 g.
- Cholesterol: 7 mg.
- Sugar: 8 g.
- Protein: 2 g.
- Total Fat: 2 g.
- Sodium: 105 mg.

93. Garlic Brussels Sprout Chips

Preparation time: 5 Minutes
Cooking time: 10 Minutes
Servings: 4
Ingredients
- About 15 Brussels sprouts
- 1 Tbsp. extra-virgin olive oil
- ½ tsp. garlic powder, or more to taste
- ¼ tsp. ground pepper
- ⅛ tsp. salt

Directions
1. Set the oven to 400°F for preheating.
2. Make 4 cups of brussels sprouts, removing enough of its outer leaves. In a large bowl, place the Brussels sprouts and add oil, garlic powder, pepper and salt. Massage the leaves gently using clean hands until thoroughly coated with the oil mixture. On a rimmed baking sheet, spread on the coated leaves in a single layer.
3. Roast for about 10 minutes until the leaves turn brown and sound crispy when tapped.

Nutrition
- Calories: 43
- Saturated Fat: 1 g.
- Total Carbohydrate: 2 g.
- Protein: 1 g.
- Total Fat: 4 g.
- Sodium: 79 g.
- Fiber: 1 g.
- Cholesterol: 0 mg.
- Sugar: 1 g.

94. Grapefruit Mint Chicken

Preparation time: 5 Minutes
Cooking time: 25 Minutes
Servings: 4

Ingredients
- 4 boneless, skinless chicken breasts (1-1 ¼ lb. total), trimmed
- Salt freshly ground pepper
- 1 Tbsp. extra-virgin olive oil, divided
- ¼ cup finely chopped shallots
- ¼ tsp. crushed red pepper
- ½ cup reduced-sodium chicken broth
- ½ cup ruby-red grapefruit juice
- 2 Tbsp. chopped fresh mint, divided

Directions
1. Season chicken breasts with salt and pepper. Set aside.
2. Heat a pan with the oil, when hot add the shallots, red pepper and cook until fragrant. Slowly add chicken broth and grapefuit. Cook until it thickens, then add seasoned chicken.
3. Serve warm and top with fresh mint.

Nutrition
- Calories: 181
- Saturated Fat: 1 g.
- Fiber: 0 g.
- Cholesterol: 63 mg.
- Total Carbohydrate: 6 g.
- Protein: 24 g.
- Total Fat: 6 g.
- Sodium: 199 mg.
- Sugar: 0 g.

95. Green Veggie Bowl With Chicken Lemon Tahini Dressing

Preparation time: 30 Minutes
Cooking time: 10 Minutes
Servings: 4

Ingredients

- ¼ cup tahini
- ¼ cup cold water plus 2 tablespoons, divided
- ¼ cup lemon juice
- ½ tsp. minced garlic plus 2 sliced garlic cloves, divided
- ¼ tsp. ground cumin
- ½ tsp. kosher salt, divided
- 1 cup green beans
- 1 small broccoli crown
- 4 (4 oz.) chicken cutlets, trimmed
- ¼ tsp. ground pepper
- 2 Tbsp. extra-virgin olive oil, divided
- ½ large red onion, sliced
- 4 cups thinly sliced kale
- 2 cups cooked brown rice
- ¼ cup chopped fresh cilantro

Directions

1. In a small bowl, whisk ¼ cup water and tahini until smooth. Add ¼ tsp. of salt, lemon juice, cumin, and minced garlic. Whisk to blend and reserve.
2. Trim the green beans and slice them in half. Cut the broccoli into florets. Measure one cup (save the remaining for another use).
3. Season the chicken with pepper and the remaining ¼ tsp. of salt. Over medium heat, heat one Tbsp. of oil in a large cast-iron skillet. Place in the chicken and let it cook for 3–5 minutes on each side until an instant-read thermometer reads 160°F. Place into a clean cutting board and keep it warm by tenting with a foil.
4. Wipe the pan out and pour in the remaining 1 tbsp. of oil. Add onion and let it cook while stirring once in a while, for 2 minutes. Add the sliced garlic and let it cook for 30 seconds.

Then place in the green beans and broccoli. Cook while stirring from time to time, for 2 minutes. Mix in the kale and pour in the remaining 2 tbsps. of water. Cover the pan and steam for 1 to 2 minutes until the veggies are tender-crisp.
5. Cut the chicken.
6. To serve, split the veggies and rice into four bowls and place the chicken on top. Drizzle with the reserved dressing and then sprinkle with cilantro.

Nutrition
- Calories: 452
- Total Fat: 18 g.
- Saturated Fat: 2 g.
- Cholesterol: 65 mg.
- Total Carbohydrate: 42 g.
- Sugar: 3 g.
- Protein: 35 g.
- Sodium: 361 mg.
- Fiber: 5 g.

Chapter 13: Drinks

96. Avocado Blueberry Smoothie

Preparation time: 5 minutes
Cooking time: 0 minutes
Servings: 1
Ingredients

- 1 tsp. chia seeds
- ½ cup unsweetened coconut milk
- 1 avocado
- ½ cup blueberries

Directions

1. Put all the fixings listed in the blender and blend until smooth and creamy.
2. Serve immediately and enjoy it.

Nutrition

- Calories: 389
- Fat: 34.6 g.
- Carbs: 20.7 g.
- Protein: 4.8 g.
- Fiber: 0 g.

97. Vegan Blueberry Smoothie

Preparation time: 5 minutes
Cooking time: 0 minutes
Servings: 2
Ingredients

- 2 cups blueberries
- 1 Tbsp. hemp seeds
- 1 Tbsp. chia seeds
- 1 Tbsp. flax meal
- ⅛ tsp. orange zest, grated
- 1 cup fresh orange juice
- 1 cup unsweetened coconut milk

Directions

1. Toss all your ingredients into your blender, then process till smooth and creamy.
2. Serve immediately.

Nutrition

- Calories: 212
- Fat: 6.6 g.
- Carbs: 36.9 g.
- Protein: 5.2 g.
- Fiber: 0 g.

98. Berry Peach Smoothie

Preparation time: 5 minutes
Cooking time: 0 minutes
Servings: 2
Ingredients
- 1 cup coconut water
- 1 Tbsp. hemp seeds
- 1 Tbsp. agave
- ½ cup strawberries
- ½ cup blueberries
- ½ cup cherries
- ½ cup peaches

Directions
1. Toss all your berries and other fixings into your blender, then process until smooth and creamy.
2. Serve immediately.

Nutrition
- Calories: 117
- Fat: 2.5 g.
- Carbs: 22.5 g.
- Protein: 3.5 g.
- Fiber: 0 g.

99. Cantaloupe Blackberry Smoothie

Preparation time: 5 minutes
Cooking time: 0 minutes
Servings: 2
Ingredients

- 1 cup coconut milk yogurt
- ½ cup blackberries
- 2 cups fresh cantaloupe
- 1 banana

Directions

1. Toss the cantaloupe and other elements into your blender, then process till smooth.
2. Serve and enjoy.

Nutrition

- Calories: 160
- Fat: 4.5 g.
- Carbs: 33.7 g.
- Protein: 1.8 g.
- Fiber: 0 g.

100. Cantaloupe Kale Smoothie

Preparation time: 5 minutes
Cooking time: 0 minutes
Servings: 2
Ingredients
- 8 oz. water
- 1 orange, peeled
- 3 cups kale, chopped
- 1 banana, peeled
- 2 cups cantaloupe, chopped
- 1 zucchini, chopped

Directions
- Toss all your ingredients into your blender, then process until smooth and creamy.
- Serve immediately.

Nutrition
- Calories: 203
- Fat: 0.5 g.
- Carbs: 49.2 g.
- Protein: 5.6 g.
- Fiber: 0 g.

101. Mix Berry Cantaloupe Smoothie

Preparation time: 5 minutes
Cooking time: 0 minutes
Servings: 2
Ingredients
- 1 cup alkaline water
- 2 fresh Seville orange juices
- ¼ cup fresh mint leaves
- 1 ½ cups mixed berries
- 2 cups cantaloupe

Directions
1. Toss all your ingredients into your blender, then process until smooth.
2. Serve immediately.

Nutrition
- Calories: 122
- Fat: 1 g.
- Carbs: 26.1 g.
- Protein: 2.4 g.
- Fiber: 0 g.

102. Avocado Kale Smoothie

Preparation time: 5 minutes
Cooking time: 0 minutes
Servings: 2
Ingredients
- 1 cup water
- ½ Seville orange, peeled
- 1 avocado
- 1 cucumber, peeled
- 1 cup kale
- 1 cup ice cubes

Directions
1. Toss all your ingredients into your blender, then process till smooth and creamy.
2. Serve.

Nutrition
- Calories: 160
- Fat: 13.3 g.
- Carbs: 11.6 g.
- Protein: 2.4 g.
- Fiber: 0 g.

103. Apple Kale Cucumber Smoothie

Preparation time: 5 minutes
Cooking time: 0 minutes
Servings: 2
Ingredients
- ¾ cup water
- ½ green apple, diced
- ¾ cup kale
- ½ cucumber

Directions
1. Toss all your ingredients into your blender, then process until smooth and creamy.
2. Serve.

Nutrition
- Calories: 86
- Fat: 0.5 g.
- Carbs: 21.7 g.
- Protein: 1.9 g.
- Fiber: 0 g.

104. Refreshing Cucumber Smoothie

Preparation time: 5 minutes
Cooking time: 0 minutes
Servings: 2

Ingredients

- 1 cup ice cubes
- 20 drops liquid stevia
- 2 fresh limes, peeled and halved
- 1 tsp. lime zest, grated
- 1 cucumber, chopped
- 1 avocado, pitted and peeled
- 2 cups kale
- 1 Tbsp. creamed coconut
- ¾ cup coconut water

Directions

1. Toss all your ingredients into your blender, then process until smooth and creamy.
2. Serve.

Nutrition

- Calories: 313
- Fat: 25.1 g.
- Carbs: 24.7 g.
- Protein: 4.9 g.
- Fiber: 0 g.

105. Cauliflower Veggie Smoothie

Preparation time: 5 minutes
Cooking time: 0 minutes
Servings: 2
Ingredients

- 1 zucchini, peeled and chopped
- 1 Seville orange, peeled
- 1 apple, diced
- 1 banana
- 1 cup kale
- ½ cup cauliflower

Directions

1. Toss all your ingredients into your blender, then process until smooth and creamy.
2. Serve.

Nutrition

- Calories: 71
- Fat: 0.3 g.
- Carbs: 18.3 g.
- Protein: 1.3 g.
- Fiber: 0 g.

106. Sweet Dream Strawberry Smoothie

Preparation time: 15 minutes
Cooking time: 0 minutes
Servings: 1
Ingredients

- 5 strawberries
- 3 dates, pits eliminated
- 2 burro bananas or small bananas
- Spring water to make 32 oz. smoothie

Directions

1. Peel off the skin of the bananas.
2. Wash the dates and strawberries.
3. Add bananas, dates and strawberries to a blender jar.
4. Add water and mix. Continue to add sufficient water to get up to be a 32-oz. smoothie.

Nutrition

- Calories: 282
- Fat: 11 g.
- Carbs: 4 g.
- Protein: 7 g.

107. Apple Blueberry Smoothie

Preparation time: 15 minutes
Cooking time: 0 minutes
Servings: 1
Ingredients
- ½ apple
- 1 date
- ½ cup blueberries
- ½ cup sparkling callaloo
- 1 Tbsp. hemp seeds
- 1 Tbsp. sesame seeds
- 2 cups sparkling soft-jelly coconut water
- ½ Tbsp. bromide plus powder

Directions
1. Mix all the fixings in a high-speed blender and enjoy!

Nutrition
- Calories: 167.4
- Fat: 6.4 g.
- Carbs: 22.5 g.
- Protein: 6.7 g.

108. Avocado Mixed Smoothie

Preparation time: 15 minutes
Cooking time: 0
Servings: 1
Ingredients
- 1 cup water
- 1 oz. blueberries
- 1 pear, chopped
- ¼ avocado, pitted
- ¼ cup cooked quinoa

Directions
1. Blend all fixings in a high-speed blender and enjoy!

Nutrition
- Calories: 187
- Fat: 21 g.
- Carbohydrates: 29 g.
- Protein: 11 g.

109. Peach Berry Smoothie

Preparation time: 15 minutes
Cooking time: 0
Servings: 1
Ingredients
- ½ cup frozen peaches
- ½ cup frozen blueberries
- ½ cup frozen cherries
- ½ cup frozen strawberries
- 1 Tbsp. sea moss gel
- 1 Tbsp. hemp seeds
- 1 Tbsp. coconut water
- 1 Tbsp. agave

Directions
1. Put all the above fixings in a blender and blend for 1 minute.
2. If the combination is too thick, add an extra ¼ cup of coconut water and blend for another 20 secs.
3. Enjoy your peach berry smoothie!

Nutrition
- Calories: 170
- Fat: 0 g.
- Carbohydrates: 43 g.
- Protein: 0 g.

110. Irish Sea Moss Smoothie

Preparation time: 15 minutes
Cooking time: 0
Servings: 1
Ingredients

- 2 oz. whole, wild sea moss, soaked
- 2 cups spring water

Directions

1. To prepare Irish Sea Moss Smoothie, use 2 whole and wild sea mosses
2. Carefully wash away any sand and debris
3. Do a final wash and chop up longer ones to safeguard your blender's blade
4. Add your sea moss and 2 cups of spring water to blend in the blender
5. Put in a jar and refrigerate. This smoothie can last for many weeks
6. Enjoy your delicious smoothie

Nutrition

- Calories: 220
- Fat: 3 g.
- Carbohydrates: 45 g.
- Protein: 2 g.

111. Strawberry Banana Smoothie

Preparation time: 15 minutes
Cooking time: 0
Servings: 1-2
Ingredients
- 2 cups Hemp milk
- 4 bananas
- 8 oz. strawberry
- ¾ cup dates
- 1 Tbsp. agave

Directions
1. For making this delicious smoothie, you need to place the strawberries and dates in a high-speed blender.
2. Blend them for 1 minute or 2 or until they are slightly broken down.
3. After that, add the banana along with the hemp milk and agave.
4. Blend them for 2–3 minutes or until combined well.
5. Enjoy.

Nutrition
- Calories: 148
- Fat: 2 g.
- Carbohydrates: 21 g.
- Protein: 1 g.

112. Green Monster Smoothie

Preparation time: 15 minutes
Cooking time: 0
Servings: 1

Ingredients
- ½ avocado, diced
- ½ mango, diced
- 2–3 dates, pitted
- 1 Tbsp. Soursop pulp
- 1 bunch rainbow kale, leaves torn
- ½ cup coconut water

Directions
1. For making this smoothie, place all the ingredients in a high-speed blender and blend them for 2–3 minutes or until everything comes together and smooth.
2. Transfer the mixture to a serving glass and serve it with ice cubes if you desire to take it cold.

Nutrition
- Calories: 179.4
- Fat: 2.3 g.
- Carbohydrates: 36.8 g.
- Protein: 6.8 g.

113. Apple Smoothie

Preparation time: 15 minutes
Cooking time: 0
Servings: 2
Ingredients

- 2 cups apple juice, fresh
- 2 cups ice cube
- 1 Tbsp. Sea moss
- 1 clove, grounded
- 1 Tbsp. ginger, grounded

Directions

1. To start, place all the ingredients needed to make the smoothie in a high-speed blender. Mix them for 2–3 minutes or up until you get a smooth mixture.
2. Serve and enjoy.

Nutrition

- Calories: 431.5
- Fat: 10.8 g.
- Carbohydrates: 53.1 g.
- Protein: 38.4 g.

114. Apple Cucumber Smoothie

Preparation time: 15 minutes
Cooking time: 0
Servings: 1
Ingredients
- 1 large to medium size sliced cucumber.
- 1 large cubed apple.
- 1 large sliced bell pepper.
- 6 seeded dates (rinsed).
- 6 large strawberries.
- 5 sliced tomatoes (rinsed).
- ½–1 cupful water.

Directions
1. Combine the whole recipe and blend very well until smooth.
2. Wow! The first-day breakfast is settled; enjoy.

Nutrition
- Calories: 65
- Carb: 57 g.
- Protein: 2 g.
- Fat: 4 g.

115. Multiple Berries Smoothie

Preparation time: 15 minutes
Cooking time: 0
Servings: 1
Ingredients
- ¼ cupful blueberries.
- ¼ cupful strawberries.
- ¼ cupful raspberries.
- 1 large banana (peeled and sliced).
- Agave syrup, as desired.
- ½ cupful water.

Directions
1. Transfer the water into the blender.
2. Add the remaining ingredients and blend until smooth.

I really love this smoothie because it is very sweet without adding sugar, and the color is also inviting.

Nutrition
- Calories: 210
- Carbohydrates: 55 g.
- Sodium: 20 mg.

116. Kale Smoothie

Preparation time: 10 minutes
Cooking time: 0 minutes
Servings: 2

Ingredients
- 10 kale leaves
- 5 bananas, peeled and cut into chunks
- 2 pears, chopped
- 5 Tbsp. almond butter
- 5 cups almond milk

Directions
1. In your blender, mix the kale with the bananas, pears, almond butter and almond milk.
2. Pulse well, divide into glasses and serve. Enjoy!

Nutrition
- Calories: 267
- Fat: 11 g.
- Protein: 7 g.
- Carbs: 15 g.
- Fiber: 7 g.

117. Raspberry Smoothie

Preparation time: 10 minutes
Cooking time: 0 minutes
Servings: 2
Ingredients
- 1 avocado, pitted and peeled
- ¾ cup raspberry juice
- ¾ cup orange juice
- ½ cup raspberries

Directions
1. In your blender, mix the avocado with the raspberry juice, orange juice and raspberries.
2. Pulse well, divide into 2 glasses and serve. Enjoy!

Nutrition
- Calories: 125
- Fat: 11 g.
- Protein: 3 g.
- Carbs: 9 g.
- Fiber: 7 g.

118. Pineapple Smoothie

Preparation time: 10 minutes
Cooking time: 0 minutes
Servings: 2
Ingredients
- 1 cup coconut water
- 1 orange, peeled and cut into quarters
- 1 ½ cups pineapple chunks
- 1 Tbsp. fresh grated ginger
- 1 tsp. chia seeds
- 1 tsp. turmeric powder
- A pinch black pepper

Directions
1. In your blender, mix the coconut water with the orange, pineapple, ginger, chia seeds, turmeric and black pepper.
2. Pulse well, pour into a glass.
3. Serve for breakfast. Enjoy!

Nutrition
- Calories: 151
- Fat: 2 g.
- Protein: 4 g.
- Carbs: 12 g.
- Fiber: 6 g.

119. Beet Smoothie

Preparation time: 10 minutes
Cooking time: 0 minutes
Servings: 2
Ingredients
- 10 oz. almond milk, unsweetened
- 2 beets, peeled and quartered
- ½ banana, peeled and frozen
- ½ cup cherries, pitted
- 1 tbsp. almond butter

Directions
1. In your blender, mix the milk with the beets, banana, cherries, and butter.
2. Pulse well, pour into glasses and serve. Enjoy!

Nutrition
- Calories: 165
- Fat: 5 g.
- Protein: 5 g.
- Carbs: 22 g.
- Fiber: 6 g.

120. Blueberry Smoothie

Preparation time: 10 minutes
Cooking time: 0 minutes
Servings: 1
Ingredients
- 1 banana, peeled
- 2 handfuls baby spinach
- 1 Tbsp. almond butter
- ½ cup blueberries
- ¼ tsp. ground cinnamon
- 1 tsp. maca powder
- ½ cup water
- ½ cup almond milk, unsweetened

Directions
1. In your blender, mix the spinach with the banana, blueberries, almond butter, cinnamon, maca powder, water, and milk.
2. Pulse well, pour into a glass and serve. Enjoy!

Nutrition:
- Calories: 341
- Fat: 12 g.
- Protein: 10 g.
- Carbs: 54 g.
- Fiber: 12 g.

Chapter 14: Prenatal Exercise

Have you ever seen a pregnant lady and thought, "Wow! How does she do that?" The answer is exercise, and it can increase the health of both mother and child. It's an easy fix to maintain weight before pregnancy or to maximize fitness during pregnancy. But there are so many opinions about what type of exercise is best for a pregnant woman, which can be frustrating. There are 2 types: aerobic exercise (e.g., jogging) or strength training (e.g., lifting weights). If you are trying to increase muscle despite the fact that you are pregnant, it can be challenging because your uterus is in such close proximity to your spine that heavyweights may injure the baby inside of you.

Is It Safe to Exercise When You Are Pregnant?

The main reason for exercise during a woman's pregnancy is to maintain health and strength. It is not recommended to do anything that could cause trauma or stress on the baby or herself, so if you are not sure about an exercise, don't do it. In fact, many doctors will advise their patients not to perform specific exercises such as yoga or horseback riding if there is a chance of falling down.
Drinking plenty of water can be beneficial as well when pregnant. While it may be easier said than done, allowing yourself time to rest and relax is equally important during pregnancy.

Benefits of Exercise During Pregnancy

Exercise during pregnancy is good for you. It can help to increase muscle tone and strength in the last trimester, and it may help to prevent complications such as high blood pressure, constipation, gestational diabetes, or some other pregnancy-related problems. During pregnancy, women may not feel like exercising because they are feeling a change in their bodies. They may also be concerned about causing harm to the baby inside them. However, doing strength training exercises can help increase muscle tone and strength, which helps prevent problems with blood pressure, gestational diabetes, or constipation. Strength training may also help with the prevention of pre-eclampsia (a risk for the mother's health if she becomes pregnant again within a year or has had a history of this condition).

Substances are used to diagnose gestational diabetes and high blood pressure. Blood pressure is lowered when necessary to keep sudden changes in blood pressure under control. If the mother tests high for her blood sugar, then she may be instructed by her doctor to exercise more often than usual to help bring it down.

Toning exercises are great for increasing muscle strength and tone. They also help promote relaxation without being too intense or overly fatiguing. Some of these exercises include light jogging swimming walking or cycling.

Recommended Exercise

Here are some of the most commonly recommended exercises during pregnancy, as well as some that are not recommended:

Aerobic exercise: High-impact aerobic exercises such as jogging are not usually recommended during pregnancy because the baby is likely to get injured from falling too hard on the ground. However, low-impact exercises such as walking swimming, and cycling are good choices.

How often to do it: If you have been exercising before you got pregnant, it is a good idea to continue that exercise routine throughout your pregnancy if you enjoy doing it. If you have not exercised before and want to start during your pregnancy, talk with your doctor about a good workout plan for you. You may have to reduce the frequency and intensity of exercise as your pregnancy progresses.

Exercises to Avoid

Avoid exercises that involve lying flat on your back for any length of time. This includes the following:

- Abdominal exercises while lying flat on your back
- Supine pelvic tilts done in a propped-up position (on the bed, for example)

Conclusion

Gestational Diabetes is a type of diabetes that is diagnosed during pregnancy and occurs due to hormonal changes in the mother.
Gestational Diabetes can be caused by many factors but is often triggered by obesity and genetics. Women who are obese or have a family history of diabetes are at greater risk for Gestational Diabetes than women who are not obese.
As those hormones mentioned earlier cause glucose levels to become high, this increases the demand for insulin production from the pancreas. Problems with insulin production may lead to gestational diabetes development because your body does not produce enough insulin for your blood sugar levels before it becomes too dangerous and unmanageable.
As we end this book, here are some points to remember about Gestational Diabetes:

- Gestational Diabetes can occur in a pregnant mother, but the mother does not necessarily have to have Type 1 or Type 2 Diabetes.
- Gestational Diabetes is caused by hormonal changes and is temporary.
- If Gestational Diabetes is not treated, a woman could face serious health issues for both her and her child if it were to go untreated during pregnancy.
- Gestational diabetes occurs mainly in women who are obese or have a family history of diabetes (genetics).
- There are many symptoms of Gestational Diabetes such as thirst, passing urine more frequently, headaches and blurred vision, fatigue, increased hunger/appetite, and unexplained weight loss for no reason at all.
- Gestational Diabetes is not a lifelong disease. It usually resolves itself within the first 6 months postpartum and does not cause any long-term damage to health.
- Gestational Diabetes can be managed with diet/exercise and insulin or oral medications such as Metformin, Lispro, and Repaglinide (Prandin).
- Gestational Diabetes can be prevented by finding out if you have the gene for diabetes or are at risk for it by following basic lifestyle advice such as eating healthy foods, exercising regularly, having a healthy weight before pregnancy, and getting proper prenatal care during pregnancy.
- If Gestational Diabetes does arise, there are many treatment options to help manage the blood sugar levels.
- Gestational Diabetes is only a temporary condition that resolves itself with proper intervention.

- Gestational Diabetes does not cause long-term damage to health, so let's prevent its occurrence before it arises. This would help prevent you from having to live with any complications that might arise from its development if it were not handled properly and/or managed properly by a doctor or regular healthcare provider.
- Eating healthy foods and exercising regularly will help prevent the occurrence of Gestational Diabetes during pregnancy.
- Proper prenatal care will also help prevent the occurrence of Gestational Diabetes during pregnancy.
- If you have a family history of diabetes (genetics) or are at risk for developing diabetes, be sure to maintain proper lifestyle habits before getting pregnant to ensure a healthy pregnancy for you and your child.
- If you are already pregnant, it is important to talk about your risk with your doctor so that you can go about preventing it (through diet/exercise) and managing it properly if it does occur (through insulin or oral medications).

I hope that this book will help you understand how we can prevent, manage, and possibly even cure Gestational Diabetes.

Made in the USA
Coppell, TX
05 October 2021